Praise for

"Creating a life you love with of might feel like a tough ask of anyone who is childless. If that impossible for you at this time, and you're uncertain of what is next, Lana Manikowski offers to walk beside you. Her book, *So Now What?*, is a great springboard to finding support that works for you. Lana offers real-life examples from her own experiences and, as fans of *The "So Now What?" Podcast* will know, it's said with authenticity and empathy. Lana's approach follows a pathway from self-reflection to dealing with a world that can feel overwhelming with tried and tested approaches based on her learning. I wish I'd had this book to hand after my experiences of failed IVF and miscarriages."
—Berenice Howard-Smith, MA, co-founder and director of the Full Stop Community CIC and co-presenter of *The Full Stop Podcast* (thefullstoppod.com)

"If you're facing the heartbreak of not being able to create the family you dreamed of, Lana's beautiful book will provide both solidarity and solutions for your "now what?" You are not alone. There is hope. This is an inspirational read for anyone facing a life childless not by choice."
—Jessica Hepburn, author of *The Pursuit of Motherhood*, *21 Miles*, and *Save Me from The Waves*

"In her deeply kind and reassuring manner, Lana talks about things I've never heard someone else say about unexplained infertility and childlessness—and I've literally written a book about it! This is an invaluable addition to your shelf and a real help to living a good life on your terms. A glorious and comforting "it's not just me!" hug in a book."
—Kat Brown, editor of *No One Talks About This Stuff*, journalist and author, Scorpio, owner of over-dramatic animals

"Whilst Lana acknowledges the grief of infertility and the struggles she has faced, her encouragement and enthusiasm help to lift you and see your life from a different perspective. She provides simple exercises to change ingrained negative thought patterns and inspires you to take steps that will create a more positive future. Lana isn't just a coach; she's a friend who gently guides you toward finding happiness, enjoyment, and contentment as a childless woman."
—Stephanie Joy Phillips, founder, World Childless Week

"Lana Manikowski's *So Now What?* is an essential guide to the often not-talked-about side of infertility. *So Now What?* offers a blueprint for navigating the unknown and unexpected world of childlessness by focusing on your relationship with yourself, with others, and with the world around you. Lana excels in empowering you to truly thrive after infertility. As a fertility doctor, I'm thankful to have *So Now What?* as a resource for all my patients who are looking for support after moving on from fertility treatments."
—Natalie Crawford, MD, double board-certified OBGYN/REI and host of the *As a Woman* podcast

So Now What?

So Now What?

CREATE A LIFE YOU LOVE
WITHOUT THE CHILDREN
YOU ALWAYS DREAMED OF

LANA MANIKOWSKI

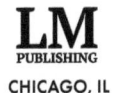

CHICAGO, IL

LM Publishing, Chicago, IL
Copyright © 2025 by Lana Manikowski. All rights reserved.

No part of this publication may be reproduced, stored in a retrieval system, or transmitted in any form or by any means (electronic, mechanical, photocopying, recording, or otherwise) without the written permission of the author and publisher.

Library of Congress Control Number 2025902401
Paperback ISBN: 979-8-9921927-0-4
eBook ISBN: 979-8-9921927-1-1
Book cover and interior design by Christina Thiele

Editorial production by KN Literary Arts

*To all the women who dreamed of motherhood but
were never able to achieve it.
And to my husband, Jack, who's been my rock through all of it.*

Contents

Foreword ... xi
Introduction ... 1

PART 1: Your Relationship with Yourself

1: Finding Your Turning Point After Your Treatment Journey Ends ... 8
2: What Do You Believe ... 16
3: Forgiving Your Thoughts and Creating New Ones ... 22
4: The Difference Between Thoughts and Facts ... 30
5: Responding to Your Reactions and Feelings ... 38
6: Knowing the Difference Between Self-Compassion and Self-Pity ... 44
7: Believe, Feel, Act ... 50
8: Planning Your Thinking ... 56
9: Learning Not to Fear Change ... 62
10: Grieving What Might Have Been and Redefining Your Future ... 70
11: Who Are You Now? Who Do You Want to Become? ... 76
12: Identifying Your Desires and Creating New Goals ... 84
13: Choosing to Love Your Life After Infertility and Redefining Your Worth ... 90

PART 2: Your Relationship with Others

14: Avoiding Isolation and Strengthening Existing Connections ... 98
15: Addressing Loneliness and Finding New Friendships ... 108
16: Acknowledging Change in Ongoing Relationships ... 114
17: The Solution to the Drama ... 120

18: The Distinction Between Addressing Your Needs and Being Selfish	128
19: You Can Always Adopt! And Other Clueless Things People Say	134
20: Will My Marriage Be Enough?	140
21: Telling Your Story and Educating Others	146

PART 3: Your Relationship with Holidays and Events

22: Happy Holidays . . . Maybe?	154
23: Halloween and Christmas	160
24: Mother's Day	166
25: Father's Day	174
26: Birthdays and New Year's	180
27: Baby Shower Invites	188
28: Locations Associated with High Emotion	194
29: Owning Your Time	200

Resources	211
About the Author	213

Foreword

In my decades of supporting, advocating for, and connecting childless women globally, I've been privileged to be the private vault of many thousands of personal stories. In doing so, I've noticed issues that many struggle with, and that often straddle cultures, situations, and ages. And thus, I am deeply heartened to say that in this kind, compassionate, but above all practical guide to a childless life after infertility, Lana explores many of those themes.

Whether it's rebuilding your shattered relationship with your body and dreams after being blindsided by infertility, charting a new course within existing relationships with friends and family while also refreshing your friendship circle, or compassionately discerning the difference between cutting yourself some slack while grieving or avoiding the painful work of healing from the heartbreak of thwarted motherhood, Lana has it covered.

In particular, her sections on dealing with "difficult questions" about our parental status and reframing how to manage family-focused holidays, including Halloween, Christmas, New Year's and Mother's Day, feel innovative, attainable, and worth the guided effort she shares, step-by-step. Even though I am many years into my own recovery from unexplained infertility, I found new insights here.

Like so many of us, Lana's childlessness dragged her through a crushing dark night of the soul, and her readers are extremely fortunate that she emerged from that "cocoon of grief" with a new understanding of herself not just as someone who had longed to be a mother, but as a human being of intrinsic value and with an abundance of love to share in other ways—along with a zeal for supporting other women childless after infertility to find *their* way back to meaningful lives too.

Whilst this book focuses on the experience of heterosexual, partnered women who've experienced fertility treatments, there is wisdom here for all of us unexpectedly living a life without children. Upbeat, focused, grounded, and compassionate, Lana's book is a warm, precise and elegantly crafted addition to the growing canon of literature for the childless not by choice.

Jody Day, psychotherapist, founder of Gateway Women (gateway-women.com) and author of *Living the Life Unexpected: How to Find Hope, Meaning and a Fulfilling Future without Children.*

Introduction

Hello, beautiful, I'm so glad you're here! Whether you've come to this book through *The "So Now What?" Podcast* or are new to my community of powerful women who have survived infertility, welcome! If we were in person, I'd give you the biggest hug ever because . . . I'm a hugger.

Before getting into the refreshing perspective this book will offer around being childless not by choice, I want to tell you that I see you. You belong here. I am in admiration of all you have navigated during your infertility journey.[1] Being unable to achieve your dream of motherhood can feel so unfair, and we're often left to figure it out with little support.

That all will end here, because you've found me. I'm going to show you how to thrive after infertility, how to find purpose and meaning, and—most importantly—how to recapture the vibrancy and zest for life you once felt. It's still there; it's attainable.

I know because I've been where you are.

In my teen years I'd daydream about how my life would unfold: how many children I'd have, the man I'd marry and—of course—the traits that would make him a great father. I dreamed of a house in the suburbs, a white picket fence, and an expansive backyard with a swing set for the kids. A lot of thinking went into what my life as a mother would look like, but one thought never occurred to me—what if I never became a mom?

I have always been a woman who knows what she wants

---

[1] Throughout this book I use both the terms *fertility journey* and *infertility journey*. For me, both are valid and describe different stages of my overall experience. When I was actively in the midst of treatments, I thought of it as my fertility journey—because I was seeking fertility. Eventually, knowing I would never become a mother, I began thinking of my overall journey as one of infertility.

and figures out how to attain it. My enjoyment in life went unchecked until the age of thirty-seven, when I was diagnosed with unexplained infertility. I went into solution mode, which meant that my husband and I endured several rounds of IUI and IVF at multiple clinics across the country. We invested hundreds of thousands of dollars in treatment and travel, not to mention the emotional and mental drain of timed intercourse, varied treatment protocols, and perfectly administered trigger shots. I was a walking pin cushion suffering endless blood draws and a constantly bruised stomach from FOLLISTIM and MENOPUR injections. Despite the dedication, despite the torture, despite the investment, my seven-year journey through fertility treatments ended without a child, and I was blindsided. Everything I had hoped for was out of reach. Everything I had desired was not going to happen. I felt cheated and totally unprepared for my childless life.

In the months and years that followed, the vibrance of hope I once felt drained from me, only to be replaced by shame and misplaced anger. Fate had not given me a child, while so many others around me enjoyed parenthood. I avoided social gatherings where I was questioned about my childlessness and was offered unwanted advice about things I should be trying to become a mom. Shame was pervasive: for choosing not to adopt, for both how my body had failed me and how it looked, for not knowing how to move forward.

My once carefree and purpose-filled life became filled with disappointment. I was mentally, emotionally, and physically exhausted and couldn't recognize who I'd become. I see now that it was a difficult but critical period I needed to move through in order to make the next discovery—that I was missing out on more than just motherhood; I was missing out on life.

I needed to allow myself the time to mourn the mother I thought I would become. I chose to forgive my body for not doing what I thought it was designed to do. I decided that my grief was valid—even if what I was grieving was a dream.

Once I allowed myself to mourn my inability to create a child, it was time to thrive again. Craving more, I decided to discover my meaning and feel fulfilled without the children I thought I'd have. I wanted to be present and contribute to the loving and affectionate partnership I had with my husband. I wanted to feel connected to friends and family and navigate through difficult conversations with them regarding my infertility. I wanted to feel proud of the woman I was, the amazing things I already had accomplished—and still could—in my life.

It may be hard to believe right now, but you are not the worst-case scenario. In this book, I'll show you how to move past where you are now and capitalize on where you're going. I'll share my personal stories of not only the darkest moments, but also how I rose above them to recognize all the value I carry not as a mother, but as myself. I encourage you to keep a journal and complete what I call *paper thinking*—journaling prompts you will find in each chapter—as these are a key part of this process. You will learn how to claim your future, one that brings the fulfillment, purpose, and meaning you are deserving of. I've done it. Thousands of my clients have done it. You can too.

Do I still have bad days? Hell, yeah! The world is filled with triggers when you are childless not by choice: first day of school social media posts, baby shower invitations, and—of course—the endless ad campaigns that come along with Mother's Day. I've discovered how to navigate the world and these situations as a childless person by learning the key to living my life deliberately and with purpose.

That choice is available to you as well. I felt so alone during my infertility journey, and I looked for a community of women who understood what I was going through. I couldn't find one, so I created one. *The "So Now What?" Podcast*, this book, and becoming a certified life coach have all contributed to a life filled with meaning and purpose. Whatever your path toward that goal looks like, I'm here to help you achieve it.

I'm so glad you've joined me in this mission to believe that your life is just as abundant, meaningful, and purposeful as anyone else's. Together we can support each other as we wake up every day choosing the life we want to live—while also recognizing that the bad days will come, and we will love ourselves then too. We are women who will not judge ourselves for what we don't have, but will take credit for what we have created and what we will continue to do. When we believe in ourselves and support one another, we can all lead deliberate and meaningful lives.

XOXO
Lana

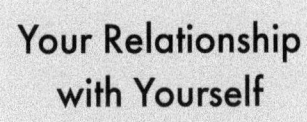

Your Relationship with Yourself

PART 1
—

1

Finding Your Turning Point After Your Treatment Journey Ends

Congratulations! You have taken a pivotal step toward transforming yourself by picking up this book. Whatever brought you here, you have decided you're ready, yearning, and deserving of more. I'll help you find clarity again while learning to thrive and discovering your purpose even though things didn't turn out as you had hoped. I know it may feel impossible, but it isn't. When my dreams came to a screeching halt, no one was there to assure me my life still had meaning. I didn't have awareness of the things you'll find in this book—things that are easily available to anyone who wants to create the life of their dreams.

The day I got "the call" from our clinic, I was away from home on a business trip in Minnesota. I wasn't expecting to hear the most devastating news I'd ever receive while I was away from my support system. The results from the genetic testing of my last frozen embryo were in; the doctor left a voice mail, warning me he was going to deliver sensitive information, and I should hang up now if I wanted to listen at another time. I'd waited months for this news, so I allowed the message to play. In that moment my life changed forever.

My only frozen embryo had trisomy 16, a chromosomal abnormality that would never result in a viable pregnancy. The message ended with, "I'm sorry, Lana. I know how badly you and Jack wanted this." I was shattered. Over the past seven years there had always been a glimmer of hope, a chance that *this* time it would work. It was finally over. My dream of becoming a biological mother was gone.

I was in shock. I needed to get away from my colleagues and find somewhere to fall apart. I found myself tucked at the end of a dark corridor in our corporate headquarters, sobbing, mourning the children I'd always wanted, the mother I deserved to be, and the future I had dreamed of. It had all been taken from me, and there was no solace. A female custodian came upon me in the depths of despair, and in my halting Spanish, I explained why I was crying. She gently put her hand on my back and said, "He will take care of you."

I'll never know the woman's name, but she was the only person present with me in the darkest moment of my life—a perfect stranger, someone whose path crossed mine exactly when I needed her. Years later, I still think of her and how she served a critical purpose: to beckon me forward out of that dark place—literally. She will never know the memory I have of her etched in my brain and the place she holds in my heart. I doubt she remembers me, and I'm certain she never considers her presence in that moment with a woman she didn't know as part of her purpose—but it most definitely was.

While it took time for me to realize it, my encounter with that woman played a role in helping me form the three pillars that are the core of my teaching methodology. Understanding the impact of these three pillars will help you create a life you love without the children you always thought you would have.

The Three Pillars

Body Image

Not only did my relationship with my purpose suffer after my diagnosis of unexplained infertility, but my thoughts and feelings about my body did too. Wrapped up with my belief that my purpose in life was to be a mother, was the belief that my body had a job: to create a child. It didn't, and I came to feel that my body had failed me, that it was broken, that it couldn't do what it was genetically designed to do.

For years after my fertility treatments ended, I continued to attribute my weight gain and change in appearance to the medications and the treatment process itself. While weight gain is a known side effect of these treatments, the truth was more complicated. I carried this explanation with me as a way to shield myself from deeper truths.

Whenever I encountered people I hadn't seen in a while, I'd feel the need to preemptively explain my appearance. I'd say things like, "Oh, I've gained weight because of fertility treatments," as if I needed to justify looking different. It was easier to blame the medications than to face reality: I stopped caring about my body because I felt so let down by it.

As someone who had always been fit and took pride in having a "good figure," it was hard to accept this new reality. I was embarrassed by how I had let myself go. I didn't want people to think I was okay with how I looked, but I also wasn't ready to do the work of reconnecting with my body. Saying my weight gain was because of treatments felt safer than admitting I was struggling to forgive my body and see it as worthy of care.

The truth is, I had given up on my body because I was grieving what it didn't give me, and I felt like it had betrayed me. Acknowledging that I gained weight was a way of recognizing just how hard everything I went through was. But forgiving my body and learning to care for it again was an even bigger step, one I didn't realize I needed to take at the time.

That all changed when I encountered Corinne Crabtree, founder of the No BS Weight Loss Program, and host of the podcast *Losing 100 Pounds with Corinne*. Corinne not only taught me how to lose my extra weight, but she also became a mentor and was instrumental in my decision to become a certified life coach myself.

One of the most important things Corinne taught me was that I could stop believing the narrative that my body was broken. Would I give birth to a child? No, but my body could do so many other things. Much like my purpose did not have to be tied to one thing, neither did my body. I could still be strong; I could still be proud. I could still love my body. It will be with me until the end of my life, and yours will too. Carrying around something you despise will make you tired and resentful.

Love your body; love yourself.

We'll talk more in later chapters about ways to work toward a future self that you can have confidence in, a future self that you can love. We'll learn about how to create habits that will rebuild your relationship with your body, as well as how to identify some habits you may have picked up along your journey that will only continue to erode your thoughts and feelings concerning your body.

Relationships with Others

Throughout my journey, I put on strong armor, not wanting to show the world my vulnerability. I kept my fertility treatments a secret at work for fear of being overlooked for advancement opportunities. Engaging with friends who became pregnant or had children was complex; spending time with friends or family who might inquire about my fertility treatments and my next steps was too. Now that my treatments were over, the constant contact and calls from my fertility clinic ceased. I had never felt more alone.

I pulled back from the world, my husband, friends and family, and surrounded myself in a cocoon of my own grief, believing that the rest of my life would be a slow, meaningless march toward death. I eventually came to realize that I was missing out on an abundant, available life—if only I would reach out and take it.

We'll be talking a lot about our relationships with others throughout this book. This includes work colleagues, your spouse or partner, and family and friends you want to hold on to—and those you might choose to let go of—as well as the ones you've yet to encounter. I can teach you how to navigate difficult conversations, truly enjoy the good times, and find meaning and purpose in your connection with others.

Owning Your Time

When I lost the dream of becoming a mother, I had to redefine my identity as well as what the rest of my life would look like. I had imagined a world where I participated in classroom parties, carted kids to practices and lessons, a world of packed evenings helping with homework and mornings making breakfast before the bus came. With one phone call, that was all gone, and I was left staring down the rest of my life, a void of time with nothing as meaningful as motherhood to fill it with.

Discovering purpose and meaning comes in a variety of ways that we will explore in this book. There were many avenues that helped me build a life that is fulfilling. From career and community involvement to developing new skills and devoting myself to a lifetime of learning, I have found the path toward a plentiful life.

These three foundational areas of focus were instrumental in transforming me from the lost and broken person I was to the strong and fulfilled woman I am today. Just like my coaching program, this book is structured around these core pillars. Part 1 reflects not only body image but also mental and emotional health by covering situations and instances in daily life that revolve around your relationship with yourself. Part 2 focuses on your relationships with others and how to maintain healthy connections with the people around you. Part 3 concerns your time, both personal and specific dates on the calendar (such as holidays and events) that many women who are childless not by choice find difficult. Moving forward, we'll explore how these areas of focus are implemented throughout my teachings and how they can help you to thrive after infertility.

2

What Do You Believe?

There are so many thoughts and feelings wrapped up in my fertility journey, and I'm confident the same is true for you. For a time, our lives were dedicated to creating a new one—and it didn't happen for us. A word that kept coming up during my treatments, whether as a test result, a diagnosis, or outcome of a cycle, was: *failed*. Implantation had failed. This was a failed cycle. I was a failed fertility patient. The reiteration of such a jarring word clung to me, invading my perception of myself and who I was as a woman. My body failed me. I failed to conceive. I failed as a woman.

The feeling of failure clouded my perception of what I was capable of, and I hit an all-time low when I was told my only frozen embryo wasn't viable for implantation. In that instant it was clear I had done everything wrong; my time, energy, and money had been for nothing. I had cheated my husband out of fatherhood; my in-laws wouldn't be grandparents. I believed I would die alone in a nursing home, that everyone pitied me, and I was the worst-case scenario. Most crushingly, I believed that I had lost the chance to lead a fulfilling life of meaning and purpose because my dream of being a mother had been taken from me.

Sound familiar?

So many of us harbor these beliefs; they are common. What isn't common is questioning them, realizing that we can change *who* we are by understanding who we *believe* we are. Through time and careful practice, I learned how to call bullshit on the rinse-and-repeat cycle of believing in my own failure, and I started to redefine my life. I've helped so many of my clients do the same: finding purpose through careful work and thoughtful self-introspection. You are no different. There is absolutely no reason you can't create the life of your dreams without the children you thought you'd have.

Let me break down the concept of what a belief is as I learned from one of my beloved teachers, Abraham Hicks. A belief is a thought you keep thinking—which means that when a thought is repeated frequently and accepted as true, it becomes a belief that shapes how you perceive yourself and what goes on around you.

The first step is to notice what you've been believing about yourself. It may sound simplistic, but the most important part of this process was recognizing what I had been thinking about myself on my fertility journey. I never knew questioning the beliefs I held about myself was an option. The word *failure* had been used so often to describe me clinically that I latched on to it as part of my identity. This may be the case for you as well, and that feeling of being a failure can leach out into other areas of your existence. The beliefs of what you're capable of start to diminish. You may even become unrecognizable to yourself.

I had a client who interviewed for a promotion at work and didn't get it. Being childless after fertility treatments, the disappointment hit her all the harder. Together, we worked through the impact of being passed over for this promotion and uncovered that being labeled as a failure during her IVF treatments had carried over into other parts of her life—and she believed it. Not receiving the promotion was, for her, further proof that she was a failure, not only at being a mother but in her career as well. Her confidence in what she was capable of started to diminish as her brain bought into the word *failure* to describe herself. Any time things didn't work out the way she had hoped, she believed it was her own fault—she was doing it wrong, and she had failed.

Your beliefs create your future. When you discover the ability to identify your beliefs, you will see where they are taking you, and you can decide if you want to continue your journey with them. You can create new beliefs that will write the story of your future so you can live the purposeful and meaningful life we are all entitled to. As long as my client clung to the belief that she was a failure, she feared taking steps to upgrade her life. Why try for another promotion or apply for a new job? Why bother making new friends or attempting a new hobby? She's a failure, after all. Best to avoid further disappointment by not trying anymore.

Luckily, I'm trained to help my clients. I was once on the same failure train and emerged on the other side, so I was able to guide her to the realization that just as easily as these thoughts had entered her life, they could be ushered right back out. She could call BS on these beliefs that weren't getting her to where she wanted to go. It may sound incredibly foreign, but it's the key to separating yourself from a belief that you have held for a long time, one that your brain has decided is a fact.

We create a codependency with our beliefs, partly because we've never questioned them, but also because it's easy to get comfortable with where we are. Change is scary, and when you're the only person who can facilitate it, sometimes staying right where you are—even if you're miserable—sounds better than trying to navigate unknown waters to create something different. I know I'm asking you to do something that seems like a stretch, especially if you've felt paralyzed by the outcome of your treatment for as long as you have. But are you willing to deny yourself the chance to create the future you want simply because exploring new beliefs feels like a challenge?

It might sound difficult, but it is the key to your freedom! How do I know? Because I was where you are. I allowed myself to believe so much that wasn't true about me because I was classified as a "failed fertility patient." I am also a strong, resourceful woman who is proud of the journey I went on, even if my result wasn't motherhood. My experience was painful, and it will never leave me. There was a time when all I wanted to do was put it behind me, block out that part of my life where I had failed.

Like my client, that feeling of failure loomed inside me until I faced it, questioned it, and realized there was another way to define myself because of that experience. I endured physical pain, repetitive ultrasounds, endless blood draws and injections. My bruised stomach and arms were not symbols of my failure, but evidence of the strength I had shown and the commitment I made to myself and my husband to try to meet our parenthood goals. I am also keenly aware of my resourcefulness, such as when all the local pharmacies were out of medication, and I was able to locate meds for a trigger shot at 3:45 a.m. By identifying my beliefs about myself and questioning them, I now see I'm not a woman who had failed, but one who earned a right to feel pride in her strength and determination.

I no longer believe the "failed" clinical terminology written in my chart, what my brain accepted as the truth. I no longer believe others were judging me and my efforts or that they viewed me only as an object of pity. I used the very tools I teach my clients to discover that I could choose a different belief, a new outcome, a better future, and that all those things were available to me if I was willing to believe on purpose.

Believing on purpose starts with noticing your beliefs, and it's a great opportunity to introduce you to what I call *paper thinking*. When I was first asked to write down my thoughts and feelings, I balked. It felt like a silly activity—after all, I know my thoughts. What's the point in writing them down? Especially when they're not kind or attractive; I'd be ashamed and embarrassed if someone ever read them!

If you're feeling the same way right now, I get it! But give it a chance, and you'll discover that there is a real relief in getting your thoughts out of your brain and onto paper—you might even realize how hard you've been on yourself when you see it in writing. Paper thinking is a transformative experience, and I urge you to give it a chance. We'll start slowly, with some simple prompts to help you identify your beliefs and question them.

When you're ready, take time to sit with yourself and your journal. Really begin to think about what you believe about yourself. It may be uncomfortable to hear what you come up with, and that's okay. No one is listening but the person who needs to hear it—you. Let go of judgments and write for your eyes only as you answer the following questions.

- What do I believe about myself?
- What do I believe about my future?
- How does this belief make me feel?
- Is it a feeling I want to feel?
- What do I *want* to believe?

Once you uncover the answers to these questions—even though they may not be rosy—you will be on the path toward a new future, one where you determine what you believe about yourself, who you are, and what you deserve. In the next chapter we'll talk about taking these answers and using them to create new beliefs that will give you the tools to create a fulfilled, meaningful life after infertility.

3

Forgiving Your Thoughts and Creating New Ones

'm so glad you're settling in with me on this journey. As you make your way through this book, my words may evoke memories of some of the hardest, most challenging days, months, and probably years of your life. The memories may still be raw, but in this chapter, I'm going to help you create an understanding of your past that is likely very different from the perspective you view it from now. Although it was painful, your past has offered you experiences that can help you step into a life that better reflects who you truly are—a woman deserving of a life you love. Before you start thinking that's impossible after what you've been through, know that most of my clients come to me feeling disappointed, defeated, and marginalized because motherhood isn't on their résumé. They are wrestling with thoughts about how they were cheated and beliefs about what should have gone differently. They believe that life has treated them unfairly.

They have yet to learn the connection between thoughts and feelings—and that *how* you feel is directly related to the thoughts you are thinking about yourself. Your opinion of yourself—and what you are capable of—is often based on things you've maneuvered through in your past and how you've shown up in your life. For example, prior to my diagnosis of unexplained infertility, I often thought of myself as a strong, hard-working, successful, goal-oriented woman who rarely came up against things she couldn't maneuver around. I felt confident and secure, able to tackle most obstacles in my path, because my thoughts about me were generally pretty favorable. If I ran into a roadblock, my inner monologue would sound something like this: *Come on, Lana—you can do this! What's the worst that'll happen? I'll figure it out. I know what I'll try!*

Don't be fooled. I had bad days and times when things didn't work out as I anticipated. But my past had taught me that if I stumbled, I'd surely catch myself; I knew how to get back on my feet and plow forward. Even in challenging times, I could rely on my brain to back me up, to remind me that I'd dealt with hard things before, managed them, and moved on. But all that self-confidence and belief in myself went to shit when my fertility journey started. Cycle after failed cycle, a firm belief grew inside me that I was failing as a woman—only to be confirmed again and again. Here I was with a problem I couldn't solve, an issue I couldn't fix. I carried such a sense of shame that I couldn't do what I needed to in order to get pregnant. As the conviction that I was a failure rooted in my mind, I no longer recognized myself.

After my diagnosis, my brain turned on me, and my thoughts became my enemies, bombarding me with negative, shameful sentences that began to erode the person I had always been. Some of those might sound terribly familiar to you: *This is my fault. I shouldn't have waited so long to try to have kids. I cheated my husband out of fatherhood. My body failed me. What's my purpose without children? I'm going to die old and alone in a nursing home. I no longer fit in with my friends who have children.*

My mindset, and the foundational beliefs I held about myself, changed dramatically. I no longer faced problems with the confidence that I could handle them. My inability to get pregnant kept me from trying new things, setting new goals, or advancing in the workplace for fear that I wouldn't be able to do that either. I attached myself so completely to the word *failure* that I believed there was little I was good at anymore. I didn't recognize myself any longer and had no idea how to rectify it. Not being able to have a child meant I wasn't actually the resourceful woman I had always believed I was.

I stopped thriving. I stopped finding joy in small places and meaning in other areas because I couldn't figure out how to have a child. The life I dreamed of didn't turn out as planned, but that didn't mean that the life I was living didn't carry great value. I just couldn't see it because of the constant barrage of my thoughts. Before I could move forward and create a life I truly loved, I had to form a different relationship with my thoughts around who I was and how I showed up during my fertility treatments. I chose to separate the outcome of that snippet in time from my overarching belief about myself and my feelings of worthiness. Learning how to do that created so much freedom in my life and my future.

Noticing the thoughts you've been having about yourself and the journey you have been on will allow you to understand why you are feeling the way you do. Reciprocally, you may notice how you are feeling and recognize a thought that keeps playing in your brain, causing you to feel the way you do.

Once you get that synced up, it's imperative you forgive yourself for being so hard on yourself. You have gone through something traumatic; your dreams and goals aren't turning out like you thought they would. You are grieving the life you thought you were supposed to have, so it only makes sense that you are going to have negative thoughts—about yourself, about your future, even about others. You question why someone else could get pregnant when you couldn't, and then you beat yourself up for not being happy for them. I'm here to tell you, that's okay. Those are normal reactions, and you are not alone in having them. Extend yourself some compassion; show some love for yourself. This is all new to you. You are navigating a new normal, a new normal in which you are childless.

You not being able to have a child doesn't mean you won't be good at anything anymore. It's like your brain says, *Hey you! Fertility treatments didn't work for you so why would you bother trying to lose that weight you gained or interview for a new job? What makes you think you'll fit in with the moms in your circle if you don't have kids?* When you read that it sounds ridiculous, right? But that's the pattern of thinking your brain has adopted. And the best news is, I have the tools to teach you how to unravel all that nonsense.

Your thoughts hold incredible power. Not being able to have a child doesn't define you—it's the meaning you attach to it through your thoughts that shapes how you feel. You might find yourself thinking that your life will never feel abundant or meaningful or struggling with the belief that this isn't where you imagined you'd be. Those feelings are valid, and it's okay to sit with them.

But when you're ready, you can gently explore the possibility of what comes next. It's not about dismissing your pain or forcing yourself to move on—it's about opening the door to new possibilities and finding a way forward that feels true and fulfilling for you. If you're not going to be a mom, what is it you want to be? What legacy might you leave behind?

A lot of infertile women struggle because they have accepted society's tired, old, and outdated thoughts: that a woman who is not a mother is not fully a woman or they believe others feel sorry for them, which makes them feel pitied. Those are *other* people's thoughts and beliefs. But now that you know your thoughts are up to you, things will change. It might sound simplistic or too easy, but the truth is that you get to decide what you want to believe. No one can tell you what to believe about yourself or what you are capable of. That is your thought to choose, one that you can hold inside and nurture as it grows. No one has to know, agree with, or approve of what thoughts you are working on believing in that beautiful brain of yours. Creating your own thoughts—thoughts about you that feel good, make you proud, and bring you joy—are available right this second. A thought is just a sentence, and you get to create what words form that sentence. Wouldn't it be beautiful to choose a thought that is representative of who you want to be? For example, replace *nothing I try ever works out* with *I'm willing to see what happens if I try this*.

Your thoughts and beliefs about yourself cause you to feel a certain way, and how you feel will propel you to—or not to—take specific actions in your life. A chain of cause and effect from thoughts to actions happens, and the results of who you are, and what you're going to be, go back to the thoughts you are thinking. The thoughts you think about yourself will ultimately create a life you love. You can believe differently about your life and future if you're not going to be a mom. You can create a life you love without the children you thought you would have. Prepare to see positive changes unfold when you welcome this new tool into your life.

To help you get started, let's do some more paper thinking. Grab your journal and your thoughts and allow yourself to notice what's coming up for you. Do not censor it, do not judge it—it is truly a mirror into your brain. You can write down whatever it is you're thinking and feeling and extend compassion toward yourself. Remind yourself that you've been through something

incredibly hard, and it's perfectly normal for you to feel these things. Ask yourself:
- What do I think about my life?
- How do I feel when I think about my life without children?
- What do I *wish I could believe* about myself?
- What would it be like to feel that way?

Sit down with your answers to those last two questions and allow yourself to imagine that unfolding for you. Imagine how much lighter life would be if you started to believe that was possible for you. This chapter taught you the first steps in creating possibilities for your future—all the things you want to accomplish, all the places you can go, all the people you can meet. Through this paper-thinking exercise, you have already started to redefine who you will become and the purpose you will fulfill.

Never stop believing that you can discover your meaning!

4

The Difference Between Thoughts and Facts

A large part of learning how to shake those icky thoughts and starting to believe new ones begins with allowing yourself to daydream a bit. Try it with me—close your eyes and imagine yourself free of all the heaviness that has accumulated. Imagine life feeling easy again. A path toward attaining that future version of you lies in knowing the difference between thoughts and facts. If you're anything like me, you've created a story about yourself—the story of your infertility journey. Already, in these first few chapters, you've started redefining that story by no longer attaching the word *failure* as a self-description. In this chapter, you'll discover how to recognize the different interpretations of your story and if the story you've been telling yourself is actually true.

Let's start with what the truth is in the first place. The story you've been believing about yourself is simply a collection of *thoughts* you've continued to think, likely gathered from your upbringing, education, or the circle around you. You never really questioned them because that's just how it is. Just because those thoughts may seem true does not make them *facts*. Facts are indisputable circumstances. For example, let's take a person's age and make a statement: Sheila is forty-five years old. That's a fact because Sheila was born forty-five years ago.

When you tell yourself your own story—or relay it to others—you are constructing a narrative in a way that *seems* accurate to you, that seems to be true. But that story is a gathering of your thoughts, which are simply interpretations of your experiences. The key here is that you have the opportunity to choose how to interpret them. The only place the truth about yourself exists is in your own mind, and you have the power to choose that truth, which will then become the truth in your day-to-day life. This is where all your agency is, all your choice, all your power.

An event or circumstance is neutral and non-emotional, something that everyone can agree is true. You don't have any sort of reaction to a circumstance until you have a thought about it. Sheila being forty-five years old is a fact that has no emotions attached to it until Sheila has a thought about it, which may be influenced by society, family, or cultural traditions. Sheila may think of herself as being behind the eight ball, that she should have life figured out by now. On the other hand, maybe Sheila comes from a family that celebrates strong women. She may think that this is the phase in her life where all the learned experiences, financial stability, and tools she has developed over time will take her to the next level. If that's the emotional reaction Sheila chooses to attach to being forty-five, her entire outlook on her age is different.

Here's an example that will hit a little closer to home. When my reproductive endocrinologist shared that my frozen embryo had been tested and had trisomy 16, I had a series of thoughts. The *fact* that the embryo had trisomy 16 carried no emotional weight for me until I became aware of it. The embryo had trisomy 16 from the moment it fertilized, but I had no clue. I thought it was my miracle embaby. It wasn't until I knew the results of the test that the thought became *my dream of motherhood is gone forever*. My thoughts changed; the fact that the embryo had trisomy 16 remained the same.

Someone else may have had the same experience but felt grateful they had the information and didn't need to suffer through a transfer that would end in a miscarriage. A circumstance or fact means nothing until we have a thought about it, at which point we choose how to interpret it, and that choice becomes a truth we believe about ourselves.

As a certified life coach, I often have clients who view their circumstances as a result of feelings. They often want to change their circumstances, not realizing that facts are not what is causing their emotional distress. Facts are neutral; what causes pain is our thoughts about them. Over time, we can choose to think differently. There is more than one way to think about things that happen, but sometimes your brain will have a knee-jerk reaction of negativity because you have always assumed the negatives about yourself to be true. What goes on in your mind creates the experiences of your life.

Why does this happen? It might sound counterintuitive, but that's your brain at work, trying to keep you safe. The function of the human brain for thousands of years has been to identify danger and avoid it in order to maintain survival. Your brain cycles every fact through a filter based on your past experiences, which creates a neural pathway—an actual shortcut in your brain—so that you can react to danger more quickly. Most of us aren't living in the wild, stalked by tigers on a daily basis, but our brain still goes into survival mode to protect us from things that might not be life-threatening but are distressing nonetheless.

After your fertility treatments ended, you may have spent years of your life listening to a negative soundtrack inside of your head, one that sings out that you are a failure, that your life will lack purpose, that your future will be lonely because you don't have kids. Those neural pathways are well worn, like a canyon where water has flowed. Your thoughts—much like water—will follow the path of least resistance.

It may sound like I'm asking you to simply believe a more

positive thought and it will make everything better, but you have to dig deeper to facilitate change. You need to understand *why* you want to think differently—and that's where envisioning your future self is tremendously helpful. Your future self is leading a life where her infertility isn't a daily weight, an emotional drain, a touchstone for her brain to return to, reminding her of her inadequacy around every corner. How did she manage that? How is she thinking in order to believe these things about herself?

It's very difficult to let go of the negatives you have been assuming are true. As complex as your brain is, it likes repetition and simplicity, so creating new thoughts is going to force your brain to work harder. You have to relearn the very act of thinking in order to identify those patterns and create new ones.

Working on your awareness of those tired stories and perceptions will help you sift the facts from your thoughts and consciously teach your brain to attach a new story to the same facts. One way to approach this is to stay focused on the present and on your future self. It's much more fun to create thoughts that are future-focused on your success and where you're going rather than relying on your brain to provide answers that are based on the past, the origin point of your negative thought cycles.

This takes daily, deliberate practice. Each day I want you to listen for thoughts you have about yourself, your body, and your infertility journey. Even just catching one icky thought a day teaches your brain to start recognizing that not everything you think is automatically true. When you practice identifying what the facts really are versus your thoughts about them, you give yourself the gift of looking at your life from a neutral place.

When you spend time with the facts, you will have the opportunity to look at the situation without judging yourself.

Most of the time you'll discover that you have cobbled together a lot of painful thoughts over words that someone else said, or to the outcome of a cycle, to create a negative story. But that story is in your past, and it has nothing to do with how you could be showing up in your own life today and tomorrow. You have the power to give yourself the gift of choosing differently, choosing what thoughts you will have about the facts.

I know it's a lot of heavy lifting and sorting out facts from thoughts can feel like brain-breaking work, especially when your own mind wants to stay where it's comfortable—with the old story, the one that is holding you down and keeping you back. Luckily, I've learned that your best thought work will happen when you write things out, so let's return to some paper thinking.

Take some time to sit down and actually hear your own thoughts. Or, if you catch a thought during the day, don't just wish it away or forget about it. Write it down on a Post-it, text it to yourself, or jot it down in the notes app on your phone. Record it somewhere so that you can reflect on it later. Once you have identified your thoughts, sit down with a piece of paper and write your answers to these intentional, targeted questions.

- How does this thought make me feel?
- Why do I want to keep thinking this?
- How does this thought inspire me toward a goal I am looking to achieve?
- What would I be feeling if I thought differently?
- Why do I want to feel that way?
- What do I wish I could think about this circumstance?

Recognize and celebrate yourself just for hearing the thoughts, even if you don't like them, or if they feel uncomfortable. Moving forward, we'll cover different ways to change your negative thoughts but being able to observe them is always the first step.

5

Responding to Your Reactions and Feelings

In previous chapters we've talked about recognizing thoughts and feelings that don't feel so great and becoming aware that you can be more connected to how you think about yourself, which will impact how you show up in your life. Now, we're going to move on to understanding why you do some of the things you do, even though they don't feel productive, make you proud, or align with the person you desire to be.

An example of this is called *buffering*—the use of external things to change how we feel internally. Our brains are wired to seek pleasure and reduce pain, and you may often find yourself looking to external things to change how you feel internally. It might offer you a respite in the moment, but when you buffer, you are not fully experiencing your emotions. Instead, you are escaping discomfort—and simultaneously escaping the opportunity to learn and grow.

Dopamine is a pleasure chemical associated with the brain's reward system. When we do something that feels good—drink a glass of wine, go shopping, eat cookies, scroll social media—our brain releases dopamine. Unfortunately, this neurotransmitter is also associated with reinforcement, which is why, once you've had one drink, or one cookie, it's almost impossible to say no to the second one. Your brain learned that this action makes you feel good and allows you to escape any discomfort you are feeling.

Today's society bombards you with instant gratification. Opportunities for pleasure are countless and easily accessible now more than ever. External pleasure providers—companies and corporations that provide us with these escapes—make a lot of money on the fact that you are going to have another drink, stay on Instagram a little longer, or buy that designer handbag.

When our brain feels pleasure, it wants more—and in our world, it's easy to get. You can play a mindless game, shop online, or hop on TikTok at any moment. When pleasure and gratification are available with no effort at all, you begin to expect that you are entitled to feel pleasure all the time. Unfortunately, all that pleasure doesn't add up to happiness. All it does is provide an escape from reality, an escape from the issues you don't want to face or fix. Even worse, there is an equal and opposite consequence when dealing with false pleasures.

Once the initial rush is gone and that bag of chips is empty, you step on the scale in the morning and reality comes rushing back in. That bag of chips may have felt like a haven when you were down, but what it really did was take you away from feeling your negative emotion—and now that emotion has come back to hit all the harder. That handbag you bought was wonderful until the credit card bill came. The hour you spent on Instagram put you behind in your work, and now stress is piling up.

Pleasure is not the same as well-being. One is fleeting; the other will give you the opportunity to gain confidence, and the more confidence you have, the more grounded you will feel. Soon you have so much more to offer the world, which will allow you to show up as an empowered, fulfilled woman. When you try to avoid your negative feelings with buffering, it's like pushing a beach ball under the surface of the water; you might be able to hold it there for a while, but it will pop back up. Instead of spending all your time holding the ball down, why not address why it's there in the first place, and take the steps to understand why it's there? Imagine what your life could be like if you didn't escape in order to cope. What is the feeling that you wanted to get away from so badly that you plowed through your snack drawer, went on a shopping spree, or lost yourself on Netflix for hours? Why not address the feeling so that you won't feel dependent on the cycle of buffering again?

The first step to saying no to your buffers is recognizing what they are, then realizing that there's nothing outside of you that could ever fix your discomfort, uneasiness, or dissatisfaction. Some of your buffers may be immediately obvious to you, others less so. A great way to identify them is to refer to what your goals for your future self are, and what may be preventing you from accomplishing them. Do you want to be more fit? Diving for the Oreos when you feel stressed won't help you achieve that. Do you want to be less stressed about finances, or maybe save for a big vacation or a new home? Buying that Gucci bag might feel insignificant, but it's chipping away at the nest egg you were hoping to use for a meaningful future purchase.

Once you've determined how you are buffering, you have three options. You can allow the urge to overwhelm you and make your goals all the more difficult to achieve. You can also deny the existence of your urge, white-knuckling your way through every moment of feeling the need to buffer—which, ultimately, will only create more stress. The third option will be the most beneficial: allow the urge to be there, simply observe it, and choose not to act upon it. The grace and love you show yourself when you allow yourself to be curious about the feeling that pushes you to buffer will be some of the greatest work you do.

By observing your buffering of choice, you will discover what the feeling behind it is, and the more attention you pay to the thought or feeling that triggered your buffering action, the better prepared you will be to deal with it next time. The more you are aware of what you're thinking and how it's affecting your actions each day, you'll notice the direct correlation to the results you're seeing in your life. Using this practice, you will have the ability to create a future that you love because you have the freedom and the skill to choose deliberately—to choose not to avoid negative emotions by indulging in an action that will not benefit you or help you achieve your goals.

Once you have identified how you buffer and the emotions you were trying to avoid in doing so, remember to forgive yourself. It may be hard to recognize that you ate an entire bag of Doritos because you came home to an empty house, and that felt so lonely in the moment. Recognize that you have been through something traumatic, and your coping mechanisms helped you survive until now. However, if you want to move toward the empowered future self of your dreams, you have to identify what is no longer helping you achieve your goals.

Buffering can be an uncomfortable concept to unpack because it may feel like I'm asking you to strip your life of the small things that make you happy or to abandon some elements of self-care that you have found useful in the past. However, there is a critical difference between enjoying a simple pleasure in life and turning to it repeatedly to escape your feelings. Grabbing drinks with friends because you want to spend quality time with people that you care about isn't buffering. But having those drinks at a family event because someone made a judgmental comment about your childless status is buffering because you are turning to the drinks to avoid the negative feelings their comment caused you to feel.

In the next chapter, we'll explore buffering further and discuss the key differences between self-care, self-compassion, and self-pity. Before you move on to that, take the time to sit down with your journal and do some paper thinking about your personal buffering techniques. Remember to take time to contemplate and answer honestly, without any feeling of judgment for yourself. Identifying your buffering of choice can be uncomfortable, but it's a necessary step to move forward into future growth.

- What is a feeling I wish I had less of?
- What is something I do when I feel that way?

6

Knowing the Difference Between Self-Compassion and Self-Pity

In the last chapter we talked about buffering and how to identify some of the actions you take that aren't doing you any favors. It's important to understand that having a couple of glasses of wine with friends to socially connect may be appropriate, while drinking those glasses alone because you had a bad day and want to escape your feelings is buffering. Similarly, there's a distinct difference between self-compassion and self-pity that needs to be explored to understand that some thoughts and reactions may be holding you back rather than offering you actual comfort or forgiveness. Being able to differentiate between the two can be a critical part of understanding your journey through infertility, as certain things may carry high emotional impact.

One of those things would be baby announcements.

I'm sure you've been there—the embossed envelope came in the mail; the one that you will never get to send. You opened it up to see little baby feet in pink or blue, maybe a cute verse about the little bundle of joy that's been born . . . and you feel anything but joyous. Instead of being able to celebrate this milestone in your friend's life, you feel emptiness, loss, and even worse—jealousy. Quick on the heels of that comes another feeling—shame. *What kind of person am I if I can't be happy for my friend?*

The cycle probably sounds familiar. Feeling bad about feeling bad, thinking you were cheated, then judging the person you've become. This is the shadow self-pity casts over you, holding you back and robbing your dreams by leading you into inaction. Truthfully, feeling this way is pretty common, and you are not wrong to feel cheated for what you have experienced. You have been through so much! But sitting in these feelings long term will keep you from growing through this experience. You may see yourself become bitter as you get stuck on the merry-go-round of pointing out all the ways things haven't worked out, brooding about what other people achieved so easily while you put your life on hold for umpteen years trying to create a baby.

The cycle of self-pity is particularly devastating because it may be difficult to realize you are in it. If you are stuck in a rut where you believe that life is unfair and you got the short end of the stick, it leads to someplace even worse—the possibility that you don't deserve better. Once that thought has taken root, you'll start to see evidence of it everywhere. You didn't get the promotion at work? Your self-pity track tells you, *Of course you didn't. Nothing ever works out for you. It's not that the other person was more qualified, it's because you didn't deserve it.*

Self-pity keeps you stuck, retelling the story of your suffering and the unchangeable instance of your infertility. Women in the infertility community often feel like they are the worst-case scenario of womanhood—childless. If you are constantly telling yourself that life has cheated you, that you have been robbed of ever feeling complete, that your luck is always bad, you will be led into a victim mentality, one where inaction is desirable because taking chances and trying something will only lead to failure.

The baby announcement may sit on your table for days, staring you down. A wave of emotions begins to rise—anger, sadness, frustration. How could they send this to you? Don't they know what you've been through? And now, you're left with an uncomfortable decision: How are you going to respond? Will you send a gift? Ignore it? Your mind races with questions.

You might feel like the sender is completely clueless about your pain, that they've overlooked the deep wound you carry every day. On the flip side, if you hadn't received the announcement, would that have stung even more? Would it feel like they didn't want to burden you with their joy or, worse, that they thought you were too fragile to handle it? You might imagine they see you as jealous, unable to celebrate their happiness, or that your grief might overshadow the joy they're sharing.

These thoughts and feelings can lead you to a place of self-pity—a space where you replay your story of loss, believe the worst about others' intentions, and feel isolated. It's a place where resentment takes hold and the world feels like it's moving forward while you remain stuck.

But there's another path—one of self-compassion and forward-moving energy. The key is to understand what you're feeling and allow yourself to feel it. Receiving the baby announcement isn't what's causing your pain; it's the thoughts and emotions tied to it that feel overwhelming. It's okay to feel hurt. It's okay to feel angry. But self-compassion means stepping back and acknowledging: *Of course, I feel this way. I've been through so much, and this is hard.*

Recognize the facts: You received a baby announcement. The emotions tied to it are valid and real, but they don't need to define you and magnify your childlessness. Self-compassion allows you to hold space for your grief while also choosing to not let it shame you. It's not about denying your pain but about reminding yourself that your feelings are understandable and that you can respond with kindness toward yourself. *This is hard, but I am allowed to feel what I feel. I am allowed to take the time I need.*

There is an opportunity here—not to diminish your pain or force yourself to "move on" but to offer yourself grace as you navigate this moment. You can choose to honor both your feelings and your resilience, responding in a way that aligns with your needs and your healing. It only makes sense that celebrating something you wanted so badly but couldn't have will bring up some challenging emotions for you. Normalize that feeling of self-judgment and disappointment and recognize that other women in the infertility community have had the same reaction—you are not alone. You are not a horrible monster for not immediately feeling a rush of joy for the happy new mother. Show self-compassion by noticing what you are feeling, and then normalize it. Once you've stopped judging yourself for experiencing your own emotions, you'll see a shift in the way your energy is moving. Listening to yourself and acknowledging your feelings while also recognizing that other women feel the same way will put you on an entirely different emotional trajectory.

Don't be fooled—I have challenging days. But I have learned how not to judge myself for having them, opening the door for self-compassion rather than self-pity. When I see a mother and baby connecting while they wait in the grocery checkout line or when I walk through the maternity aisle at Target and wonder what I would have looked like pregnant, that can definitely stir up emotions for me. I'm not immune to the feelings, but I tell myself that of course I feel that way, and of course I am curious about what might have been. I practice talking to myself like I would a friend who came to me for comfort. I let those things sit with me, and I feel them. Because I have learned to practice self-compassion over self-pity, I am in a much more settled place than I was when I was playing victim to my infertility.

What goes hand in hand with understanding your feelings?

You guessed it—paper thinking. When you do paper thinking, it helps you pay attention to the thoughts and feelings, the ups and downs that are part of every day. When you put that all down on paper, it will help you start to understand exactly what it is that you are feeling and what actions you take because of that feeling. The next time you find yourself stuck in a cycle of self-pity, sit down with your journal and ask yourself some questions.

- What am I thinking when I learn that someone I know is pregnant or had a baby?
- How do I want to respond to this information?
- Why is it okay if I prioritize my needs right now?

Write as much as you need, do whatever it takes to get those emotions out of you, and realize that you might feel anxious or overwhelmed as you question yourself. Allow yourself to lean into this practice and live your life, having the human experience that is yours and yours alone. It can be messy, and it is an ongoing struggle, but you are not alone. Examining these emotions is how you will get to the other side of infertility, where you are thriving and feeling fulfilled again.

7

Believe, Feel, Act

You've been doing a lot of heavy lifting in the past few chapters. You've learned about the difference between thoughts and feelings, how to recognize your thought patterns, and how to begin the process of creating new ones. Now, I'd like to introduce you to one of the most powerful tools in your toolbox—the believe, feel, act cycle. Sometimes I refer to this in my head as "big freakin' answers" because it can offer so much clarity around how you are showing up in the world. The BFA cycle can lead you to a place of awareness concerning how your beliefs impact the things you are propelled to do—or not do.

We've already established that facts don't have an emotional impact until you attach a thought to them. Because many of us are conditioned by the beliefs our families or society have established, you likely think there's no other way to look at your circumstances—it's what your brain has been conditioned to do. So, when I went through seven years of fertility treatments and wasn't able to have a child, I believed my future was going to be lonely and devoid of meaning. It's how society portrays women like me. No one taught me I had the option of believing I could create a life I loved even if my future looked different than I expected. It all makes sense now. Those old beliefs created feelings of disappointment and emptiness, which kept me in hiding and disengaged from the woman I was before infertility.

Here's another example that you may have experienced in your life—your best friend is having a baby. A strong belief about yourself is going to come hard and fast on the heels of this, and it's probably something like *life isn't fair*. That statement automatically sets you up as the victim. When you feel victimized, you may find yourself comparing all the ways you're more deserving of motherhood than she is, judging yourself and trying to think of what you did wrong, or creating reasons why this didn't happen for you. Or maybe you are believing that you're unrelatable because you are the only one in your friend group who won't be a mom, which makes you feel isolated. And when you feel isolated, you don't reach out to your crew or only begrudgingly accept invites to girls' night, looking for all the ways you believe you are being ignored in conversations.

Let me be clear. The beliefs you have are valid; your feelings are authentic to you. The way you respond to these circumstances doesn't have to be explained or justified—*you are entitled to all of this*. But know that if you don't like the way you are feeling, there are other options.

So many of us have spent our lives blaming how we feel on the world, believing that facts and situations have created our emotional reactions. Most of us have never been taught that we are in control of our emotional life. You can decide what you want to believe and then take control of your feelings. Once you realize this, you'll be able to do things that you never thought were possible, and you won't move through life believing that other people or situations have the power to make you feel bad.

After my fertility treatments failed, I blamed fate for what I believed would be my future: an empty life, devoid of purpose. Once I started paying attention to my thoughts, it was astonishing how loud and overwhelmingly dark they were. I believed that I would never love my life, I would never know love as a childless person, my failed cycles meant that something was wrong with me, and the cherry on top—I'm was also a terrible person at my core because I couldn't be happy for my friends when they got pregnant.

It's no wonder that loving my life felt so hard at that time. I was focused on all the things that didn't happen for me. I needed that time to feel the devastation. I wouldn't be where I am today if I didn't feel the immense loss and uncertainty about my life without children. But I got to a point where I didn't want to believe those stories about myself anymore or feel the way I did because of those beliefs. Luckily, I learned that there was another way. I started examining what I was believing and was able to prove this old, crappy belief system wrong. I realized that I could believe something new.

What would I rather believe? How would I like to feel? What are some of the actions I would rather take or not take when feeling this way?

Allowing yourself the space to consider these questions is important, because taking action is the hardest part. You've built up a series of beliefs and feelings about taking action too. They might look something like this: *People will judge me. I might not be good at it. I might not know how to do it. I might not do it right.* That last one hits pretty hard for me, personally. I'm a goal-oriented woman who seeks success, and in the past, I've attached the f-word—*failure*—to any action as an excuse to not even try. If you're a person who has a fear of not doing it right, I want to convince you that you are capable of taking action—even if you're not sure of the outcome.

I know you can, because you've already done it.

You had a goal of having a child and took hundreds of actions trying to make that happen. You know what it takes to put in effort. You woke up at six in the morning because you had to have blood drawn before work. You traveled for business and carried your medications in a cooler through TSA at the airport. You set an alarm for 3:00 a.m. to take a trigger shot the morning before retrieval. You said yes to round one of IUI, and maybe even round two or three. You had the hard conversations with medical professionals, your own family, and friends when they asked how things were going. If you were willing and capable of taking action in an effort to be a mom, you are equally capable of taking action for yourself and your future life, whether you have a child or not. You just have to decide when that time is right for you to believe something new about yourself. There's no timeline you have to follow, no clock you are up against. You will know when you are ready to feel better about yourself, and now you have tools to help you when that time comes.

You might have already guessed that your paper thinking for today revolves around the BFA cycle.
- What would I rather believe?
- How would I like to feel?
- What are some of the actions I would rather take or not take?

Next, do some brainstorming on actions you can take that would help move you toward that future self who is showing up in the world the way she wants to. Think of things that might move your needle even 2 percent when it comes to your thoughts and feelings. You don't have to commit to them; just write them down. Consider options that might move you into the future that you want to have, the one where you love your life, and move through each feeling energized.

You don't have to believe new things right away; that would

be extremely difficult. This is a powerful and transformative lesson, one that will not happen overnight. But you can practice seeing there's a new way of believing that will help you realize that your current beliefs aren't the only truth out there, they aren't the only option. The goal is not to feel better right away, but to achieve an understanding of your beliefs so that you can feel anything you want, on purpose. You can create evidence for yourself that you are the sole owner of your beliefs, the creator of your feelings and the one to decide what actions you do—and don't—want to take. It's given me so much freedom in my life, and I want you to know it's available to you too.

8

Planning Your Thinking

Now that you're getting your arms around the difference between thoughts and facts and becoming more adept at noticing the thoughts you've been having, you may judge yourself for some of your past thinking. You may feel like you have been doing it wrong or deliberately wallowing in self-pity in the past, but let me assure you that's not the case. Most people aren't aware that they have alternative options, so it makes total sense that you've been thinking the way you have about yourself, your body, and your future without children. Being diagnosed with infertility and maneuvering through the treatment path is likely one of the most challenging experiences you've had; thinking positive thoughts about yourself is nearly impossible.

If your encounters were anything like mine, you probably had people tell you things like, "think positively, and it will happen." This is not what I'm talking about here. You not getting pregnant had nothing to do with positive thinking. I'm talking about the way you're thinking about yourself *now* and the fulfillment of your future because you didn't have a child. When I discovered I could think something different about myself and my story, it felt like I finally had some control of my life again. The thoughts you *choose* to think about yourself are powerful.

You're building a toolbox that will allow you to perceive yourself differently and think about yourself in ways you never thought possible. Owning thoughts that make you feel like you have a say in who you are and who you desire to be will empower you. Up until you've learned this, your brain has been doing what it thought it was supposed to do—keep you alive and keep you comfortable. I know, you're probably thinking, *Yeah, but the shitty thoughts I've been thinking certainly aren't keeping me comfortable.* Let me break it down for you.

We've talked about how the human brain learns and perfects things through repetition. So if it's spent a long time believing being childless means you will be missing out on life's purpose, it's going to keep spitting thoughts like that at you when you think about your future. It's what your brain has accepted as logical; it believes that is what it's *supposed* to think. But the rational you—the one who is cognitively thinking about this now—is probably realizing that this isn't helping you. Your brain has picked up bad habits along the way and needs you to train it to start doing things differently.

Your brain creates neural pathways based on repetition. Think about athletes who train hour after hour on the same motions. They are training the body to replicate that exact form and motion so the brain fires on autopilot when they swing their golf club or precisely return a serve with their tennis racket. Those pathways are kind of like canals in the brain, and like water, thoughts will follow the path of least resistance. You've probably noticed that when you are presented with an opportunity or experience that is out of your norm, you hesitate. That's because your brain has gone into survival mode and is asking, *Hey, is this a good idea? I've never thought this way before. What if I'm totally off on my thinking here?*

It might feel like your brain is misfiring by keeping you from actively seeking new thoughts about your experiences, but what this really means is that your brain is functioning properly; it's programmed to keep things simple, to repeat what's always worked in the past. It's a lot of work to look for what's wrong, to interpret new thoughts, experiences, places, and people. And the brain isn't necessarily looking for more work to do, so it will be up to you to start training it by consciously introducing new thoughts and feelings.

The good news is that if you don't like the way your current thinking is making you feel, you can start to modify it whenever you are ready. In fact, you've already taken the first step by noticing your thoughts. Once you've developed that skill, along with knowing how to sort facts from thoughts, you can ask, *Is this an automatic thought?* Is this your brain using shorthand? Is it going for the auto-fill response instead of coming up with something new? Are those old neural pathways still wide open, making it easy for your thoughts to slip into the negative circuit? These thoughts can be so ingrained that it may not feel like a choice but a predetermined outcome.

But there is a choice.

The more attention you give to your thoughts, the more you'll see the pattern of your brain taking preventive action. Once you've realized this, you can start anticipating situations, plan your thinking, and be more deliberate with your thoughts ahead of time. As you work on this awareness, you'll get really good at boiling down your old stories to the facts and then consciously teaching your brain that it has the option to attach a new story to the same facts. When it comes to your brain attaching past lessons to future opportunities, it will try to limit you in order to keep you safe. But, as one of my mentors says, "Your past is a great teacher, but it's not a fortune-teller."

With this in mind, let's take a look at a common thought within the infertility community: *My body is broken.* You know enough about the difference between thoughts and feelings to be aware that "broken" isn't factual. Your body isn't broken, but it couldn't get pregnant. That fact probably generates a lot of triggering thoughts, which can be uncomfortable, and that is understandable. However, it's these difficult facts and thoughts that require the most work and offer the opportunities for your greatest breakthroughs.

So, your body can't get pregnant. What does that mean? In the past your brain has opened up the negative-thought neural pathways every time this thought surfaced. It wants to believe that you aren't a complete woman or you were born flawed. It likes repetition and simplicity, and these thoughts are smooth, well-worn river stones that have easily slipped down into these negative patterns before. Your brain knows this, so it will preemptively guide them in that direction once again. But—now *you* know that your brain will take this action. And guess who is in charge of your brain? You are!

I found that training your brain to consider what is possible based on the knowledge you have *now* allows you to move forward more deliberately and with so much more clarity. What *can* your body do? Does it wake up every day, willing to do the things you want it to? Could it run a 5K? Hug someone who needs support and offer them comfort in that way? Allow you to show and explore physical love with your partner? Become a vehicle for you to move through a career where you work long hours, then treat it to some well-deserved rest? Could your body be the way that you show yourself self-love and self-compassion by getting a massage, taking a spa day, or allowing that dessert to be a reward?

Your body isn't broken; it does so many amazing things. It just didn't give you the baby you thought you were supposed to have. Your future accomplishments are countless, you just need to decide what is next for you. Are there things you've thought of exploring? Have you been interested when you've heard a coworker share about classes they've taken? Start to make a list of these things. The next time the thought, *My body is broken*, surfaces in your mind, you've got an entire list of things your body can engage in doing. You've planned more favorable ways of thinking so that you can open up new, positive neural pathways. Once you get into the habit of doing this, your brain will learn that there are options, and it won't jump to negative conclusions the way it always has in the past.

Your brain has pulled together a lot of jarring thoughts over time, compiling them into the story of your suffering—the one that keeps you safe at home, not trying new things, or not allowing yourself new experiences. But your past has nothing to do with how you could be showing up in your life today. You can give yourself the gift of deciding how you want to think differently in response to some of the triggering thoughts that you've identified in your infertility journey. By doing so, you'll open up opportunities to discover the greater meaning you are creating in this world.

9

Learning Not to Fear Change

You've gone through so many emotions on this journey; a lingering sadness, stabbing guilt, and maybe even those bright, glimmering moments when you connect with another woman in the infertility community and feel like someone finally understands. In this chapter, I want to talk about an emotion that we're all familiar with: fear. It's a big emotion, one that we've all experienced in different ways, some of them quite dramatic: the moment when you slam on the brakes and just miss that fender bender, the unexpected knock on the door, the simplicity of a jump-scare in a horror flick. But fear can also work in small ways that aren't so easily pinpointed yet still have a significant impact on your life.

When my husband and I bought a house in 2015, I was in between chapters of fertility treatments. I hadn't decided whether I could put myself through the roller coaster of emotions that came with agreeing to pursue more rounds IVF, but we consciously chose this house because it allowed us room if our family were to grow. When we purchased it, I secretly identified two rooms that would make great nurseries. I envisioned myself coming home from the hospital with a baby in my arms, to this place. Even after all these years, the vision of that seems so clear.

Starting a new chapter of our lives as parents in a new home located in a neighborhood with parks and spaces to take our children for walks seemed like a dream. It had everything I wanted in terms of size and location, and I quickly went about making it mine through remodeling. I designed the most beautiful kitchen you've ever seen, picked out wallcovering, light fixtures, and draperies. It became a true nest for me, a place that held hopes and dreams—along with a vision of who I would become while living there.

That house was the setting for so many emotions. There, I prayed that saying yes to IVF again would fulfill my dream of motherhood. We hosted great parties and celebrated many occasions with family and friends. I also hit some of my deepest lows when I got the news of canceled cycles and embryos that didn't mature. There, the final call with our reproductive endocrinologist took place, confirming that our IVF journey had come to an end. My heart soared in that home; it was broken in that home. Everything I thought I would become was lost while living there, and it felt like I had very little left that could showcase my success as a woman. No successful pregnancies. No nursery to decorate. No baby to welcome home.

As time passed, my husband would throw out the idea of selling our home—something I was adamantly opposed to. Whenever we talked about it, fear bloomed inside of me, a reaction that I didn't quite comprehend at the time. Now that I understand myself much better, I know what was going on. Lost, I clung to our spacious house for validation. It felt like evidence that I had made it, that I had done something right, something people would look at and think, *Wow! Lana's got a great life*. I attached myself to things like that because there was little left I felt proud of after my fertility journey resulted in no children.

If we sold this beautiful home, I feared we'd never live in anything as impressive as that house. It was a terrible tug of war I played with myself because selling the house meant I was accepting that my journey to motherhood had come to a close. It was a reminder of what I'd never have, but I couldn't let go because I didn't know if I would ever find a beautiful home like this again. It was as if I was holding on hard to the things in my life that still felt semi-decent, clinging to something as painful as the would-be nursery simply because I believed my best days were behind me and this was as good as it could get. I couldn't create a child; but I must've done something right to have been able to afford a 5,000-square-foot home . . . right? I feared life would never be abundant again, and letting go of the evidence I created of my success felt scary as hell.

It's a slow, lurking fear, one that hangs heavy, one that you carry every day. It's a fear that you wake up to, a small voice in your head that asks each morning if the best is behind you. It's the fear of scarcity, and it's the fear of change.

It's very common for us to avoid change because we're afraid of losing what we already have. We stay where it's safe. We don't rock the boat. We get really comfortable with where we are and tell ourselves that we're happy. But what's really happening is that we keep ourselves stuck in circumstances that prevent us from moving forward in our lives. We stagnate. We don't grow. We remain where we are, and label it as being *grateful* rather than *fearful*.

For me, it was a house. Maybe for you it's a job, or a relationship, or an environment that is okay, but maybe not quite what you were hoping for. Maybe you know the possibility of something better might be out there, but that means giving up what you already have. And that's truly scary. In my case, I kept telling myself how lucky I was to have that house, but attributing it to luck meant ignoring the role I played in acquiring that house in the first place. Luck didn't deliver the keys to us; my husband and I saved and planned, worked and sacrificed to be able to afford it. And if I could accomplish that, why couldn't I let it go, safe in the knowledge that those same talents and skills were still with me, perhaps offering me the opportunity to discover something even greater?

First, I had to recognize what I was feeling, and why I was feeling fear. Then, I had to do something even harder: face the fact that I was attaching my self-worth to something tangible. I was letting the house act as a stand-in for who I was and what I had accomplished instead of just letting *myself* be that thing! As I said before, I am a strong-willed, driven woman. I've always prided myself on my work, how I show up in the world, and essentially *who I am as a person*. Why would a house be the symbol for that? Why would anything material be the symbol for that, other than my actual self?

Here's a thought I practiced holding at that time, one that gave me the fortitude to move through my fear and embark on a new journey: *No one has given me anything that I am not worthy of receiving*. I imagine that's true for you too. That doesn't mean that there haven't been wonderful people and opportunities in your life that have opened doors and that you're grateful for. But don't give all your power away to others; don't make yourself the supporting character in your own story. Everything you have, you deserve. And if you want to create something different, you can do that too. But it may mean saying goodbye.

When it was time to leave my house behind, I decided to write a letter to it, recounting all the memories that were associated with it. In truth, there were a lot of things that happened there that weren't so great. I was sitting on that sofa, in that living room, when I got the call that a cycle had been canceled. On one of my protocols, my doctor put me on Viagra, and it caused me the most excruciating leg pain I'd ever experienced, and I could only find relief by soaking in my bathtub. There were beautiful things too—moments I shared with my husband, family, and friends. The decision to pursue my life coach certification. It's where I started *The "So Now What?" Podcast* in my closet with a pair of earbuds and my laptop. It's the house where I became a dog mom to my beloved mini Aussiedoodle, Coco. Who I am becoming as a woman who is childless not by choice sprouted in that house, and I am eternally proud of that.

Writing that letter helped me recognize that all the growth, all the heartache, all the love that I felt in that house wasn't happening because I was inside those four walls. It was my mind and my feelings and the thoughts and beliefs that I took away from them that gave the house any meaning at all. In other words, it wasn't the house that provided those things—it was me. And wherever I went—for better or worse—I'd always be taking me with me!

Maybe you're thinking about changing jobs, moving, stopping fertility treatments, or ending a relationship. Many of us wait until we get to a point where we feel like we don't have any other option but to leave, and to do it out of sadness. But if you can start looking at things in your life that you desire to change, truly think about it. Give yourself a lot of love and nurturing, and you can get to a place of saying goodbye out of gratitude, with confidence in the forward growth it will bring to your life.

To begin your paper thinking on this, consider something you want to say goodbye to. It doesn't have to be earth-shattering or revolutionary. Maybe it's your IVF drawer—you know the one that has all those leftover supplements, alcohol swabs, and syringes you can't seem to part with? Or clothes in your closet that no longer fit the way you'd like them to. Maybe you want to change jobs or have a hobby or personal goal that you've been dreaming of trying but need to close one chapter before you open a new one. Start thinking about how to create a plan that doesn't feel rushed so that you can truly feel love, gratitude, and a sense of hope for what's coming next when you say goodbye to what you've outgrown.

Following, you'll find some more direct questions that will help you in your paper thinking. Again, a lot of the thoughts and feelings that come up when you're doing this work can feel embarrassing or shameful. But these answers are for you and you alone; only when you get curious about all your feelings—even the yucky ones—can you learn to say goodbye out of love and gratitude.

- What is something material in my life that I fear losing?
- What might happen if I lost that thing?
- What would it look like to choose to leave it behind because I made the conscious choice to move on?

10

Grieving What Might Have Been and Redefining Your Future

At this point, you've had some practice at catching thoughts in the moment. You're getting better at becoming aware of how they can influence your actions, and even evolve into firm beliefs that you hold about yourself—whether they are actually true or not. As we've talked about, your brain likes to follow the well-worn channels of past thoughts and beliefs, but you've been redirecting those and creating new ones. It's good practice not only for the moment, but for helping to build the whole picture of the self that you want to become.

Your current beliefs—especially the ones that you continuously beat yourself up over—are just recycled thoughts from the past. If you keep thinking them, you'll repeat the same actions and get the same results. We've talked a lot about those past thoughts. I know it's hard, but when you are ready, you have the tools to put them behind you so you can start creating from your future. What does that mean? If you want to create something new, or implement a new idea, you begin by creating a belief based on who you desire to be. So here's a big one: You have a future where you are not a mother, and you feel fulfilled, whole, and meaningful.

Does that feel like an impossible belief? It's not, but it takes the ability to allow yourself to dream again and start thinking about your future. It can feel scary to go there. It's a place you haven't been before, and it looks so different from how you thought it would. It's time to get excited about your future. Let's talk about how to do it, and we'll start by deciding to let go of the burdening feelings that have ridden alongside you for so long.

It can be difficult to imagine what you do want—because it feels like a stretch for someone who is childless after infertility—so let's look at what you don't want to be any longer.

During my fertility journey, I hit a point where I didn't want to feel disappointed anymore. I didn't want to feel like I was the only one who didn't get to experience what everyone else had, and I didn't want to think about my future as a long, empty stretch of missing out. But I had to tackle something major before I could leave all that behind me; I had to allow myself to grieve for the future I had been hoping for.

Is it possible to grieve something you never had?

Yes, it is a real thing. I'm guessing you have been going through feelings of grief but haven't given yourself the permission to acknowledge that you are grieving. Women in the infertility community aren't culturally given the opportunity to mourn for the life they thought they were supposed to have—because many people think you have to lose something tangible in order to grieve. You lose a grandparent, you grieve. If you lose a pet, you grieve. But when you lose a dream of a life you envisioned, it can be confusing. There's no language or sympathy cards that classify what you are going through—there's definitely no section in the Hallmark card aisle for women who wanted to become moms and couldn't. There's no culturally accepted way to acknowledge your loss, and no step-by-step program to guide you through it.

It's important you cut yourself some slack. Stop blaming yourself for not getting pregnant. You did all you could, including how calm you stayed, how positive you were, or how closely you followed your protocols. You invested time and money. You opened your emotions up to intense vulnerability and your body to close and nearly constant poking and prodding. You strove and sacrificed, but underneath it all, you dreamed. There's a sense of loss very few outside the infertility community can understand. You lost your dreams of creating a biological child, raising a child, growing a family, sending kids off to school, walking them down the aisle, and becoming a grandparent. Entire life experiences have been turned upside down, but there's no funeral for the vision of our future that died with that last test result.

It probably feels hard to explain the loss you feel because people are often trying to tell you how brave you are, not to give up hope, or options of things you should explore—like adoption—in order to become a parent. It's likely you feel misunderstood because those words intended to comfort you aren't what you want or need. Like you, the women I support are grieving the expectation of what life could have been, and no one has told you that is perfectly okay. No one has recognized that what you have experienced through your fertility journey is grief-worthy. It's what I've come to know as *disenfranchised grief*, which is grief that is not recognized or socially supported due to the nature of the grief.

While I was navigating my life after infertility treatments failed, I recognized the lack of tools and language for women who become unexpectedly childless not by choice. I wanted to learn how to better support the women who are grieving in our community, so I took a deep dive into grief and now have an advanced certification in grief and post-traumatic growth. I have learned so many amazing skills and useful tools and created a proven method to help women work through the heaviness they've been carrying around. Many people are aware of the classic five stages of grief, but you might not know that it is an outdated concept. Grief is not linear. Grief is not a problem you need to figure out how to solve, and in fact, it may not be resolvable. To think that you will reach a point in your life where you will never again feel sadness around your inability to become a mom is not realistic. What is realistic is the ability to feel grounded again in who you are so when these emotions come over you, you'll have all the tools you need to keep yourself feeling safe and understood.

The biggest problem for most people who feel grief is they think something has gone wrong. You feel as though your feelings aren't grief-worthy and wouldn't be understood by the people around you, so you hide them. Maybe you're like me and try to put a big act on that you're fine and unaffected by the loss of your dream of motherhood so others won't know what's going on inside. I'd like to offer you the concept that you are entitled to your grief. As human beings, we create dreams, goals, and purposes for our lives. For me, motherhood was one of the biggest dreams I had, and I'd created an entire story about what that would look like and the role I would play in it. When that narrative became an impossibility, everything I had hoped for in my future fell to the ground. It was a true loss, even if others could not perceive it that way. Infertility is a clinical diagnosis that leads to an intangible loss; no one else can see your shattered dreams and hopes. The dreams that would create your perfect life only existed inside your head, but that doesn't mean you have to suffer through grieving them alone. There are opportunities for you to process your loss, but—much like the loss of a loved one—everyone processes grief in their own way, so I encourage you to discover what works best for you.

First, acknowledge what it is you have lost. It goes beyond the inability to have children. We've lost the anticipation of what our future would look like, the possibility of achieving our own milestones along with our children as they grew and experienced life. We were expecting a life where our child's choices—what sports, which friends, that school, or this hobby—would have a hand in determining our own activities. Now, the responsibility of filling your own time weighs heavily. There is a huge loss and a burden that comes with that, and it needs to be recognized.

Second, acknowledge that the grief will never fully go away. You can move on from your past self, redefine your future, and achieve a fulfilling, meaningful life—you absolutely can. But, just like any other loss, it will tug at you when least expected and catch you off guard. The good news is that you are allowed to acknowledge that you did, in fact, lose something. Normalize the grief you feel so you can stop hiding and start showing up as you again. Being able to exist as a woman who is grieving—but not shameful of it—is powerful. Even the simple acknowledgment that they have suffered the loss of the dream of a loved one can often bring my clients to tears. The tools I teach my community exist to help them be present in their grief without feeling paralyzed by the powerlessness grief often evokes. It's something I wish I had when I was navigating my own childlessness: a person who understood, and a community I could grieve alongside, as we mourned the invisible and intangible—the death of a dream.

11

Who Are You Now?
Who Do You Want to Become?

If you're anything like me, a lot of your high school and college years were spent dreaming about what your adult life would look like. What you would do for a living, where you'd live, who you would marry, and how many children you would have. I remember paging through *Seventeen* magazine in junior high, taking quizzes about my strengths and personality traits that would help me determine what kind of partner I needed in life and what my path might be. Sure, the tick-boxes were fun, and I got some giggles out of my celebrity match-ups, but I never thought it would be so hard to figure it all out.

For a long time, being a mother was a huge part of the picture that made up my would-be adult life. When I found out that wasn't an option anymore, I was not only heartbroken—I was lost. This was a dream, yes, but it was also a goal, the next milestone on my life journey. Without that beckoning me to move forward, what could I look toward? For a long time, there was nothing to fill that void. There is no substitute for motherhood, and I made the mistake of believing that nothing could hold that amount of meaning for me. With that mentality, there was nothing to look forward to.

I'm writing this during the spring, a time in the Midwest that is full of bright, new beginnings. The days are getting longer, birds are singing, and there are buds on the trees. I've spent months living through a dark winter, surrounded by brown grass and barren branches. But overnight, something changed, and new life and purpose is springing up—literally—all around me. It's a rebirth for nature, and it's a wonderful time to talk about recreating and reinventing ourselves as women without children.

Reinventing yourself doesn't mean you are broken. It doesn't mean there is a past behind you that carries shame or that you're trying to cover up who you actually are by becoming someone new. As humans, we have an incredible ability and opportunity to rewrite our lives at any time, to use our strengths to supplement our weaknesses, and to redefine who we want to be every day, while looking in the mirror and asking ourselves who we want to be in the future. To reinvent yourself, you'll need to understand who you are today, at this very moment. A lot of people want to set new goals before they understand *why* they want to achieve them, which is a critical component. There's so much you have accomplished up to now; embrace that knowledge before you let the cloud of your childlessness stop you from believing you can figure this out.

Let's start with this: Is it possible to agree the entire purpose of your life was never only to be a mom? It may have been something you desired, but there is no one in the world who fulfills only a single purpose. Think of all the women in your life who have meant something to you—friends, teachers, coworkers, heck, the woman who does your taxes—none of them are your mother, yet they mean something to you. They fill a purpose in your life that has nothing to do with motherhood, and if they were no longer there, you would feel a loss.

The same is true for you. You were never meant to do only one thing with your life, no matter how much you wanted that thing. Now that you know you won't become a mother, it's time for you to decide the purpose you create by showing up as you each day. Here's an even bigger thought: That purpose doesn't have to be defined only by how you impact others or what role you play in the lives of other people. You can decide what purpose you want to serve *in your own life*.

You can call them goals, challenges, or purposes—but you

can find meaning in your life every day by being innately you. You can create magic for yourself in small ways by allowing for moments in the day where you are living just for yourself—with purpose. As this continues to grow, and you show up for yourself daily, notice how doing so allows you to also show up for others in ways you never realized. You might begin to think of yourself in a new way, as a different person than the woman who wanted to be a mom and defined herself only by that.

Start to ask yourself:
- What else might I be capable of?
- What are other things I want from life?
- How am I going to get those things?
- Most importantly, who will I be when I achieve all these things?

These are big questions, and they can be scary because they raise the possibility of the f-word showing up in your life again—*failure*.

As women who have been through infertility, failure carries a lot of weight with it. We associate it with outcomes of cycles and embryo transfers. Like we talked about in chapter 9, trying new things means change, and that's scary because we might fail. And if one more thing that you try doesn't work out the way you hoped, your brain might lead you down the path of believing that you are a failure . . . so maybe not trying anything new is the better solution. Your brain might talk you into staying idle so you stay safe. It tells you not to go after that thing because you can't fail at something you never try. This paralysis state carries a certain comfort with it; at least it's familiar. If you don't try anything new, you won't change, which means you can't fail.

Becoming the new version of you may seem like a stretch,

possibly even terrifying, because there's a part of you that hears someone else's story or sees someone who has rebuilt their life, and it feels like they have some special power that you probably don't have. Maybe your story feels too sad to recover from or you weren't born with whatever strength made their reinvention possible. Maybe you think that people who have this much growth and change happen in their life are just an anomaly. So instead you stay there on the sofa, with your blanket around you, and you dream of a day that you'll feel better.

I lived in that place for a long time and so have many of my clients. I decided that to move forward with my life, I had to clean up my fear of failure and the unknown. If you are ready to make the changes in your life you've been desiring, you must be willing to take charge of creating the life you want to have without children. It's a concept we aren't taught in our youth. Most of us have been told that life happens *to* us, so we move through it playing defense, not knowing that we can write the plays.

When you try something new, or head down a new path, there are going to be bumps along the way. You may get derailed or be unsure of what's next, but that's okay. Fearing failure keeps you fearful. You've been judging yourself for a long time, so it makes total sense that you don't want to put yourself anywhere near a circumstance that would elicit those feelings of doubt and self-judgment again. I have a different piece of advice. Let it come along with you—acknowledge that fear of totally sucking at something you've never done may be part of the spectrum of emotions you feel when going after something new. Recognize that it can be present, but not in charge. Acknowledge the fear when it comes up and literally speak to it.

"Hey, failure, I see you. I know you're here with me, and you're saying we've never been down this road before. What I'm trying to do is scary, and you think we should probably just turn back. But I want to try something new today, and I'm the one in the driver's seat—so put on your seatbelt, failure. Here we go!"

It might seem a bit kooky to talk to a feeling; I certainly thought so when I tried it the first time. But there was also a lightness in my stomach and a sense of calm when I acknowledged it this way—as a spirit present with me, but definitely not the one calling the shots. With that in mind, I felt more secure asking myself that harder question: What do I want from my life if it won't be motherhood?

I put together a development plan, asking myself these questions: What interests me? What are my superpowers? What am I doing when I feel most at peace? For me, my career was part of the answer. It had never been my intention to work full time; the goal had been to have children and then be a stay-at-home mom or perhaps return to work only part time. When I realized my dream of motherhood was not possible, I hit a hard slump. I'd spent seven years chasing motherhood; all my intensity and desires had gone into that, and I didn't seek out promotions or consider new career paths. Along with my life, my career was in a holding pattern: waiting for my next retrieval, praying for a healthy embryo, waiting for the month I didn't get my period. The new version of me was done with holding patterns and two-week waits. I was ready to take back the reins and explore new avenues in corporate America. I became the queen of networking, informational interviews, and stretch projects to demonstrate my leadership capabilities in the workplace. I was ready to advance. I was done waiting to see how things would end up, so I started interviewing for jobs and . . . didn't get one of them. I was always the one who was "so close" but not the final candidate.

I was disappointed, but I no longer saw my attempts for corporate advancement as failures. Instead of telling myself that I didn't get the job because I wasn't good enough, I had a new conversation. I told myself that not getting the job didn't mean I'm not good at what I do or that I'll never find another job I wanted to interview for. Maybe I didn't get it because it wasn't right for me—not that I was wrong for it. Maybe this was my sign that there was a totally different career path I was ready to explore. I had the power to decide what failure meant to me, and I decided it meant I was *trying*. It meant that if I never put myself in a situation where I had an opportunity to learn and grow, I'd never move forward, and I'd never change.

You have the power to decide who you want to be.

That version of ourselves we dreamed up all those years ago did not come to pass. But there's something else waiting to be discovered in our futures. You have the power to embrace change and redefine your relationship with failure not as something that you are incapable of, but as something that shows you are in the process of reblooming, of becoming the new, reinvented self that you determine you want to be.

For your paper thinking in this chapter, I'd like to start by simply identifying three things you want to accomplish tomorrow, strictly for yourself. Before you go to bed, write down three things you can easily do when you wake up tomorrow that will show you are serving a purpose for yourself. Anything from taking a vitamin to flossing your teeth will work!

Then ask yourself these questions:
- What is something I look forward to doing tomorrow?
- What about that thing do I like most?
- How can I find ways to do more things like this?

12

Identifying Your Desires and Creating New Goals

In the past few chapters we've talked a lot about your past, how to redirect your brain from the cycle of old thoughts, and how to start identifying as a woman who is childless. We're forward facing now, thinking about the future. In the last chapter, you thought about who you want to be. Now, we're going to take that a step further by identifying concrete desires and goals that will help you rediscover the nature of your purpose and give you the motivation to not only show up in the world, but also to do it with the drive you may have been lacking.

Your vision has been narrowed for a very long time, and all your goals and desires have been hanging on one thing—becoming a mother. Even though you cognitively know that's not possible, it can still hurt—and probably always will. But it's time to set that aside and refocus on what is possible. You've been zeroed in on one goal for so long. Time, money, emotional and physical energy, and brain space have all been entirely devoted to the goal of motherhood. That's a lot of resources! It's time to point them in another direction.

When was the last time you took an inventory of your desires and goals?

If you're anything like me, that might be difficult to answer right away. When you don't achieve your goal of motherhood, it can feel like there's a mass of dead space staring back at you when you look into the future. You thought your days would be full of packing lunches, driving kids to sports and lessons, but instead you are burdened by your free time; trying to figure out how you will fill your evenings and weekends doing something that seems meaningful and purposeful can feel overwhelming. It might be difficult to cast your situation in a new light. It might even seem callous to consider, but . . . there is a silver lining here. Once you've been through so much heartache and sadness, once you've worked your way through the weight that lies on your chest and consider the possibility that you may love your life again one day, you'll realize something amazing: You get to choose your future for yourself.

Choice has seemingly been taken from you for so long. Let's be honest—being childless wasn't your choice. But as you move forward, your time is entirely your own, and how you spend it will be your choice. You can rediscover who you are, and as you're working toward the future you want, you'll experience joy, happiness, and even stretches of contentment. At first, it might feel like self-betrayal, as if you're disrespecting the efforts and the heartache you suffered through. You're not abandoning the woman who tried so hard to get pregnant, the one who did everything she possibly could—you're offering her new hope. She'll be with you on this journey; it's impossible for her *not* to come along—she's you!

You have the ability right now to identify the life you want to move toward, even though it may not be crystal clear. If you can open your heart to the possibility that more is waiting for you, maybe something even greater than motherhood, your future will start to unfold with more clarity than you'd ever imagine. One of the ways I recreated myself was to share my story on *The "So Now What?" Podcast*. The thought was overwhelming; I hardly shared my story with the people close to me, let alone publicly on a podcast, but it was something I was determined to figure out. I did some research, asked questions, popped in a pair of earbuds, sat down on the floor of my closet, and recorded episode 1. It was scary, and my brain kept trying to talk me out of it.

Who was I to start a podcast? Who would want to listen to my story about rediscovering life after failed IVF? What if no one tuned in? Good thing I didn't listen to those little remnants of failure my brain was used to reciting, or you likely wouldn't be holding this book right now. But when I sat down on that first day, old neural floodgates opened right up and let the word *failure* slip into my thinking. That probably happened to you already, just while reading this chapter. A few ideas about things you've always wanted to try might have occurred to you, but they were immediately pushed aside because they seemed too big, too hard, too scary.

But if you manage your mind and tap into the steps of the BFA cycle, you'll be taking ownership of all the things you want to accomplish at work, at home, or in your relationships. Decide on something you want to do, try, or explore. What do you want to believe about doing that thing? How will you feel when you believe that thought? What are some things you will—or won't—do when you are feeling that way? Setting goals and believing in them enough to achieve them will certainly bring up obstacles and roadblocks, but that isn't the same thing as failure.

Why not?

Because your beliefs create your feelings, which drive your actions, and those actions ultimately produce the results you see in your life—no matter what. Good or bad, results don't just happen. Good or bad, they will move you forward through change, and if you are setting an intention instead of moving along haphazardly, you're training your brain that you want to have structure and supervision directed toward achieving your desires. Turning your energy, goals, and awareness toward the future will bring about change, both in the real world and in your brain itself. You're training your brain to be forward-focused and to leave the old patterns behind.

One of the exercises I work on with my clients is called an "I desire" statement. It allows you to start to dream again, to give yourself permission to accept that you aren't going to be a mom. So... now what? Continually wanting something you can't have will only leave you unfulfilled. You've been in a holding pattern, with one goal, for a very long time. But that desire is out of your control; the good news is that if you focus that beautiful brain of yours and all that determination you went through during infertility in a different direction, doors are going to open.

For the longest time, I held myself to the belief that my life without children could only be average, that my best days were behind me. I believed that living as a woman who is childless not by choice meant that the most I could ever expect from life might be only 80 percent of the happiness I would have had if I been able to achieve my dream of motherhood. I believed that the jigsaw puzzle of my life would always be missing a few pieces. When I realized I could reframe that story and start to desire new, different things, a new version of me started to unfold. That new version of me created a podcast, wrote this book, and founded The Other's Day Brunch. That version of me has brought together an entire community of women who now can support and connect with one another.

You do not have to feel beholden to infertility forever. Being infertile does not define who you are; it is not a scarlet letter on your chest. It's a part of your journey, and that part is over. Now, it's time to go all in on yourself and do the exploration that allows you to feel great and fulfilled again, to thrive and be the woman who is moving into her future with all the power and determination she moved into fertility treatments with. Except now, this is a choice *you're* making, not one that was made for you.

Your paper thinking for this chapter will come next, but first I want you to give yourself permission over the next few days to allow yourself to dream. Think about the vision of who you are in the future and who you would be if all obstacles were removed. Then, acknowledge there are roadblocks to this vision. Figure out what they are and how you can navigate through them. While this can be an exercise that is purely daydreaming, you might find yourself making lists about how to make this dream a reality.

Once you've let yourself dream, for your paper thinking make a list of twenty-five things that you want. They can be anything such as objects, feelings, or just a chaotic brainstorm of images. This will help you understand that there are still things you want and that you can dream again. Even thinking about these things is useful; you don't have to go out and accomplish them. Women who have been through infertility are often so trapped in the belief that they didn't get what they wanted, so they're scared to want something else, ever again.

It's time to want again, to dream again, to be driven again.

It's never too late to discover your meaning!

13

Choosing to Love Your Life After Infertility and Redefining Your Worth

I want to love my life again.

This is a yearning I commonly hear from my clients, and for years after my treatment journey ended, I dreamed of it myself. During the months and years spent navigating infertility, we were hyper-focused on one thing, one goal that ultimately, was not attainable. During that time, the idea of having a baby seemed like the golden ticket to happiness, and when it didn't become reality, the idea of being happy again felt impossible. As we talked about before, you go through a mourning period. This is an undefined length of time for you to acknowledge the weight of what you have lost and acknowledge that you are grieving—even if you didn't lose something more than a dream of how life would turn out. But now it's time to take the next step, the one where you redefine your future, reconsider your worth, and rediscover your meaning, all while learning to look at your life with a sense of love again.

It starts with deciding that you *deserve* to have a life you love. Your struggles through infertility left you battered, wondering why all these other women were allowed to have something you were denied. It can feel as if the universe sent you a very strong message that somehow, for some reason, you fell short. You weren't worthy enough. As humans, it's common to measure our worth against someone else's, always comparing, always questioning why they got something that we didn't. Battling through fertility treatments only to lose your dream can rob other accomplishments of their shine and make them feel less valuable. Other life milestones and met goals may even feel like consolation prizes compared to the triumphs and rewards you would have achieved through motherhood.

The job promotion, the dream house you just moved into,

the pet you welcomed into your family, the book you wrote, the personal record you just broke at the gym—they can all feel hollow if you set them up against the fact that you couldn't have a child. I used to believe that, because I wouldn't be a mother, life would max out at 80 percent. I didn't think I would ever find true joy or fulfillment without becoming a mom. Learning the tools that are now the foundation of my life coaching practice, I started catching those thoughts and questioning them. I would ask myself, *Why don't I feel as proud of myself as I thought I would?* Most people celebrate themselves when achieving goals and accomplishing pursuits; I just couldn't find it in me. Everything I did just seemed to fall short of the fulfillment I thought I would receive through motherhood.

I began to realize that I believed I wasn't good enough—maybe even unworthy—because I couldn't have a child. That infectious thought was seeping over into other avenues of my life, and it felt completely and utterly true. I bought into a story that society tells us: that women are supposed to reproduce. We are genetically designed to have children. When that option wasn't possible for me, I thought my best days were behind me. Coaching taught me to ask myself if I truly thought I couldn't have—or even deserve—a life I loved because I was infertile.

The truth was, I didn't think it was possible.

I'm guessing you believe a life you are absolutely in love with isn't possible for you either. It makes sense; we haven't been socialized to think that happiness is available to childless women. I decided I was ready to do some deconditioning. It was time to explore if a different story could possibly unfold for me, instead of the one that always had me feeling second best. At that juncture, I made a pivotal decision, one that has utterly transformed who I am as a person and determined my life's path. It was the beginning of my journey toward creating a life I love without the children I thought I would have.

When we perceive that motherhood should be the gold standard of our happiness, we let infertility rob us of joy by allowing it to squelch the moments of happiness we do achieve. For example, I think about the time when my husband, Jack, and I went to New York City at the last minute. We walked from our hotel in SoHo to Broadway, snagged tickets to see hunky Hugh Jackman in *The Music Man*, and scored day-of reservations at a Michelin-starred restaurant. Everything just fell into place. Before coaching, I would've chalked it up as a great experience while thinking that traveling to Disney World with the kids would have been so much better. I have had some breathtaking moments of happiness in my life that had nothing to do with motherhood, but so often a shadow would pass over them, and the happiness deflated if I allowed myself to think about how being a mom could trump a last-minute flight, a great meal, or a good show. This is *compensation*; a belief that something good came my way only to make up for the fact that I couldn't have a child. And as soon as compensation enters your feel-good moment of happiness, the moment's ruined.

As we've talked about, our brains want to keep us safe and protect us. The emotional roller coaster of fertility treatments has jolted and jostled our brains, sending them to the very heights of hope and back down again into the depths of despair when the outcomes weren't what we wanted. One way our brain tries to protect us in the aftermath of this is to *not let us fully experience happiness*. This might sound like a crazy thing for your own brain to do to you, but consider this: Your brain learns from the past, and the past has taught you that your potential hope or joy only leads to a big letdown. So, when you have good moments post-infertility, your brain arm-wrestles with the positive emotions, fearing that if you feel *too good*, it means you'll hurt more when things don't work out later.

Now, imagine retraining your brain to believe that you, a childless woman in the world, deserve happiness, not compensation. You deserve to feel good, you've created your reward, you're allowed to find joy in your days and excitement in your nights. The positive things that come your way aren't an apology from the universe for your suffering; they are good things that you have earned. How much more would you savor your joyful moments if they weren't conditional and compensatory for the amazing life having a child would have offered you?

Stop and recognize these moments when you have them. Lean in to them. What gives you joy? What are you doing when you feel that happiness or pride in yourself? Pay attention to what those things are, because they are going to inform about a future for yourself that is more accepting of the idea that you deserve happiness. In these moments, tell your brain, *I welcome this*, and it will begin to be more accepting of that fact. This will open you up to enjoying that moment and to wanting more of them. Allow yourself to experience the moments that bring you joy and positivity without poking holes in them. Welcome opportunities to celebrate yourself—the goodness, the beauty, and the fulfillment that you feel solely because you are you.

Allow yourself to stop believing that your only purpose was to be a mother. The freedom that we have as individuals to move through our life as fluid people who can change and adapt is a great gift and offers us the opportunity to discover our purpose.

No matter who you are right now, things can change for you. Things can get better, lighter, and easier, but this has to begin with your willingness to release the thought that your overarching purpose was to become a mother.

For your paper thinking today, I want you to ask yourself what it would look like for you to thrive. If you can begin to identify the things in your life that bring you fulfillment, you can use them as building blocks toward the future you who is leading a purposeful, meaningful life. Picture yourself as thriving in the future, then ask:

- Where am I?
- What am I doing?
- Who am I with?
- What surrounds me?

Your Relationships with Others

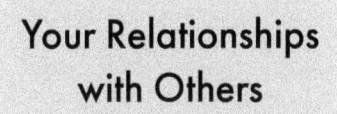

PART 2

14

Avoiding Isolation and Strengthening Existing Connections

We've been talking a lot about your relationship with the most important person in your life—yourself. There's a reason why the first part of this book is dedicated to understanding how you think about yourself: In order to make authentic connections with others, you need to have an authentic connection to yourself. Feeling connected to yourself may be a stretch right now and will likely continue to evolve. There is no itemized checklist you can go through, then say, "I'm done working on myself!" If you are looking to grow, so will your connection with yourself—it all works in tandem. It's one of the most meaningful connections that came after I decided to rediscover who I would be without children—but I didn't do it alone.

Humans are social beings, and we need a community to lead healthy, happy lives. When you're going through infertility, it can feel like no one understands your struggle, your hopes and dreams, and—eventually—the loss of those hopes and dreams. You may feel like your story is too sad to be fully expressed or that talking about it is uncomfortable not only for you, but also for the people you are sharing with. You may resort to isolation because you don't want to be the wet blanket, or you may distance yourself from others for the simple reason that being around friends and coworkers who *are* parents can be painful.

Managing your relationships with others can be a difficult path to navigate when you are childless not by choice. But giving those relationships authentic care, thought, and connection will ultimately be part of what brings you to the fulfillment of your new future and all the wonderful things you have yet to encounter. That doesn't mean you are pouring yourself into others or always being there for everyone. It may mean that you choose to let some relationships end or that you learn how to set boundaries when questions about your childlessness become too invasive. The second part of this book will help you explore different ways to maintain existing relationships and create new ones as you move into the next exciting chapter of your life!

Let's start by exploring what *connection* means to you. It might be a word that makes you think about going out, being in groups, having a girls' night, or maintaining a social calendar. That might sound exhausting or even intimidating. But connection can be whatever you want it to mean, from texting with a group of friends every day, to grabbing coffee with a coworker once a week, to just making sure that you are asking your significant other how *their* day was. A key starting block to connection is remembering that it starts with *you*, and how you are not only interacting with others but also *reacting* to them. That first critical step that you've taken to connect with yourself is key here because when you are connected to yourself, you can more genuinely connect with others.

Maybe you have that one coworker who comes in on Monday and gives everyone the updates on their weekend with their kids; from diaper changes to T-ball tournaments, their entire story is something you don't have, and it can be hard to listen to. Resentment might start to build to the point that when you see them, your first reaction is . . . *ugh*. It's an understandable feeling, and I certainly won't judge—I've been there! What I chose to acknowledge was that I was trapping myself in this story that magnified something I didn't have and putting walls up around myself to shield my feelings in the presence of people who *did* have it. My thoughts and actions were all based on lack, as if the only way I could ever feel a connection or a sense of social belonging was by being a mother . . . which I now know is simply not true.

Connections with other humans can be created in many ways. From where you went to school, to your hobbies, to sports teams, to gardening, there is common ground between you and someone who is a mother. Of course it can be annoying to listen to someone complain about their sleepless nights because the baby wouldn't settle when you'd give anything to have that in your life. But this is where all this work we are doing comes into play. This is where you catch your thoughts and acknowledge your feelings. If it's hard to listen when she gives you the play by play of her kid-centric weekend, what connection are you creating with yourself? Are you allowing yourself and your needs to be heard by you? Maybe a silent conversation reminding yourself that it's okay if this is hard to listen to, that you have relevance even if you didn't cart kids around all weekend, and most importantly, that it's not your duty to remain in a conversation that is still too raw for you to have. As women, we are often socialized to be polite, not to offend others, to put our needs last. This way of thinking often leaves us feeling violated and invisible and creates disconnection with ourselves and our stories.

As I started to create a connected relationship with myself, the connection I felt with others started to grow. As this happens for you, you'll start to realize that you don't need exact parallels with another person to create connections and have an interest in them. In fact, meeting new people who have completely different experiences than you can be exhilarating on its own. After my infertility journey I found that if I tried to force a connection with someone through common threads, it might not be fruitful. Once I had done the work on myself to feel connected to who I was as a person, meeting and connecting with someone who had completely different interests and knowledge wasn't an intimidating experience. With awareness of myself, I could connect with this person, learn something new, maybe have an engaging conversation, or possibly find a new friend.

There are plenty of relationships and connections in your life that may have been set by the wayside during your infertility journey. The pressure that comes with a cycle, the timing of shots, the care for your physical body, all took a massive amount of effort and planning. Getting together with friends took a backseat, as did maintaining connections with family. Maybe some of that drifted away because you didn't want to give updates about your infertility journey, pregnancy test results, or whether you would consider adoption if you couldn't get pregnant. That is heavy conversation that can—at times—put a wedge into lifelong relationships. It can keep you from establishing a connection with new people too.

How many kids do you have?

It's a common icebreaker question, one that most people ask without considering the possibility that you don't have any, and that even having to answer the question causes you a significant amount of stress, revealing guarded wounds right there in the middle of a social situation. The work we are doing here will free you of these "deer in headlight" circumstances so you can be in a position to respond in social situations, feeling proud of who you are and connected to the future you are creating. This is where you can start to put the self-judgment you've been feeling in the backseat.

How you respond to this inevitable question will likely take time to comfortably deliver. Planning how you answer this question—and practicing it—will be immensely helpful. In my case, I was in the habit of over-explaining myself. Instead of just answering the question, I would try to justify why I wasn't a mom, why I wasn't like everyone else, or why I hadn't chosen to adopt. Staying committed to myself and becoming secure in who I am as a woman who is not a mother has given me some options for how to handle this commonly occurring situation.

First, consider the option of just simply answering, *no*. It's two letters, one syllable. You don't have to elaborate. You don't have to apologize. You don't have to share your entire personal and painful journey. You don't have to explain yourself. Remember, it is okay not to have kids, and you did everything you could to make it happen. *Do you have kids?* The answer is no, and you can be proud of who you are right alongside that answer. There is nothing embarrassing or shameful about not being a mom.

Second, have a prepared answer. Whether you are reconnecting with an old friend who is inquiring about your current status or you have just met someone new and they've unknowingly set a bomb in your lap, being ready for the question means not only that you have an answer on hand, but that you've also done the emotional work of preparing yourself for the conversation. Simply saying, "It's not in the cards for us," or "That particular journey didn't end the way I'd hoped," are perfectly acceptable answers. There are plenty of statements that you can have ready when someone asks if you have kids or an old friend inquires about where you are now with infertility. Again, you don't have to expand on these answers. Most people will have the tact to move on from there; you don't owe anyone your story, and you aren't expected to share your pain.

It's possible that you aren't ready for the simple no or the prepared statement. There is also the chance that the person you're speaking with won't take the hint. In this case, it's more than okay for you to shift the focus, and there are plenty of polite ways to do that. "I appreciate your interest, but that's not something I'm up for chatting about," is a perfect way to let them know that this avenue of conversation isn't open for you right now.

Even better, have your own redirect ready so you can shift the focus away from children entirely. "No, I don't have children. But that means I'm able to invest a lot of my time and energy into other things I find meaningful!" My charity for homeless animals! Setting new personal goals at the gym! Repurposing old jewelry! Whatever it is that you are passionate about, you can not only signal to your conversational partner that the parenting conversation needs to be over, but there also might be another way you can connect: This is what I like. What do you like?

Another option is to have a trusted friend or family member serve as your wing person. More than likely, you've got a silent sign you use with your spouse or significant other for social situations when you are ready to leave or want a particular conversation to end. There's no reason why you can't establish this within a friend group as well. If you've got a great group of gal pals—but one ceaselessly talks about her kids—let a trusted member of the group know how this makes you feel. They can either try to redirect these conversations or create a side conversation with you at that time so you don't have to participate. This same tactic works great at family functions where you may have an aunt or cousin who always wants the update on your uterus.

You may even get to a point when you choose to take this conversation as an opportunity to educate the person asking the question. Let them know that infertility is a very real issue for a lot of women in the world. Not every woman is able to get pregnant, and adoption isn't always the answer. Being up front with someone about the very real struggle that women with infertility deal with might make them realize that starting a conversation by inquiring about kids might need to be reconsidered in the future.

However, if you're not ready to have these conversations at all, always be aware that it is perfectly acceptable for you to excuse yourself from them. If you're in a social setting like a networking event, and you're aware of a certain person who is using the child question as an icebreaker, you are not wrong to avoid them or excuse yourself to the bathroom if they enter your circle. Again, you don't owe your story to anyone, and you should never be in a situation where you feel pressure to share when you are not in an emotional place to even supply a simple answer. Maybe there will be a day when you are, but don't force yourself into it because you feel pinned against a verbal wall.

For a deeper dive into helping you get comfortable with these kinds of situations, I created a free resource, "The Top 27 Things People Say When You Are Childless (And How to Respond)," available for you to download at lanamanikowski.com/thingspeoplesay.

For your paper thinking today, think about how you would like to respond to these questions when they come your way. If you'd like to practice the simple no, do that. Make a list of other topics you'd be open to talking about with a stranger and options of how to impart knowledge around who you are in the conversation. If you're thinking about relationships that already exist with family or friends that may cause tension for you, consider who you can count on to be a buffer for you in these situations.

Whether you're thinking about new relationships or old ones, taking a step toward breaking your isolation is the next step on your journey to becoming the new you, and all the meaning and fulfillment that is waiting for you!

15

Addressing Loneliness and Finding New Friendships

When I found out I couldn't have a child, I cocooned myself in an attempt to protect myself from the outside world. There were so many reasons—pure sadness, shame, disappointment. But I also felt unrelatable, like no one could ever understand how I was feeling. There was grief, as well as judgment for myself, and dread of that suffocating, empty space in my future that was supposed to be filled by a child.

There were times I felt alone when I was surrounded by people. I'd disconnect from my true feelings and put on a front for others, as if my life was going great, as if I had emerged unscathed from my battle through infertility. I'd act interested as a coworker shared how terrible her morning sickness was. I listened as friends complained about packed weekend schedules carting kids from soccer practice to birthday parties. I'd talk about how great my life was, the new handbag I bought, or the vacation we were planning in the hopes that others would see my life as enviable.

But it was all an act to keep everyone from knowing that my heart was broken. I'd arrive home exhausted from pretending for the outside world. I didn't know who I had become and where Lana before infertility went. I had never felt so alone. I now know that the disconnection I created with the world around me was the result of the disconnection I felt for myself. I craved connection but didn't believe I could ever find it. This is how *The "So Now What?" Podcast* was born. It was an opportunity to create the connection I was seeking, and I knew if I was seeking it, my listeners probably were too. In September 2021, I recorded the first episode, not sure if anyone would even find it—but they did. My inbox began to fill up with messages from women all over the world saying, *Thank you. I didn't know anyone else felt like this.*

Beyond the podcast, so much more has come about since that time. Something I look forward to every year is The Other's Day Brunch, an annual event that takes place the day before (US) Mother's Day. It is for women who feel disconnection around Mother's Day—maybe because they don't have kids, no longer have a living mother, or have a strained relationship with a mother. I created this opportunity for women to gather, meet new friends, and feel a sense of connectivity, celebration, and love at a time that feels so unexpectedly challenging. Each year, women are elated to find perfect strangers with whom they can identify in a community of women that wants to connect and feel celebrated on a weekend that historically felt really heavy for them. This one day on the calendar can bring up so much fear and resentment for us, but now we have something else we can look forward to!

There are plenty of online options to connect with other women who know exactly what you're going through. I organize a Meetup group for women who are childfree and childless with in-person events and opportunities for women to connect with other women without children. This childless community continues to grow; new people find us every day and are excited to be welcomed to a group where they don't have to explain themselves or the size of their family. In this group and in my social media communities, women find a shared appreciation and respect for each other and their journeys, and the best part is that they are everywhere online. In the resources section of this book, you'll find listings for my Facebook group, my social media channels, as well as a more intimate offering—my signature program, Thrive After Infertility. There, I bring a carefully curated group of women together who are looking to grow beyond their infertility. It's beautiful to connect with childless women creating a life they love, without the children they thought they would have.

Of course, you might be looking to connect with new people and *not* have the conversation start with being infertile. Starting new friendships as an adult can be difficult. We all have busy schedules, and many adults have already-established social circles that can be hard to find a spot in. Like dating, it's hard enough to find someone you have something in common with and actually like—then you have to make room for them in your life. But new friendships do happen, and many of my clients have shared their methods for finding other women to connect with.

I can't drive through Chicago without seeing some sort of new workout studio—aerial yoga, hot yoga, Orangetheory, Solidcore—the list goes on. Joining a gym is good for you in so many ways. Your body will thank you, and as you continue to show up, some faces will begin to look familiar, and small talk conversations will open into something bigger. Athletic friendships can be a big part of someone's life; quite a few of my clients have joined tennis groups when someone was looking for a doubles partner. Lately, pickleball seems to be exploding, and I've participated in MUDGIRL—a muddy obstacle course event that is open to all skill levels and celebrates women.

Something else I can't drive through Chicago without seeing is someone walking their dog. As a dog mom, I'm a member of a Facebook group that has brought some great connections into my life. Dog parks are teeming not only with people who want to find a friend, but dogs too! Utilize your potential to become friends with other dog moms. Start by suggesting a playdate for your furry children and see if a friendship sparks between you and the other owner.

Volunteering is always an option. Is there something you are passionate about or a cause you'd like to lend a hand to? Showing up is the first step, and you're sure to cross paths with like-minded people. The same is true of a book club—the social glue is already built in. Check at your local library to see if they have a monthly book club or some already existing club that might be attractive to you. Libraries are social hubs for everything from gardening to tabletop gaming. There's likely something that will draw your eye, and you'll be walking into a group that shares your interests.

You might even find the key to future friends in your past! One of my clients is very active with her college alumni association. It might feel like high school was a long time ago, and you may believe you are well-rid of some classmates, but people change, and the adult version of someone you didn't exactly jibe with back then might be exactly your cup of tea now. Don't duck out of reunion invitations, or even Facebook groups, simply because you'd like to leave that all behind you.

Really not interested in reinvesting in old friends? What about friends of current friends? I can't tell you how many times I've had someone tell me that they've got a friend they just know I would totally hit it off with, but we never actually take the step of exchanging numbers or setting up a lunch date. Yes, it can feel weird to be the one initiating. You don't want to come off as creepy or weird, but in all likelihood, the person on the other end *also* has anxiety about being the one to reach out and is hoping you will.

Finally, I'm offering myself up to be your new friend! Your story is never invisible to me, and you can find me online through Facebook and Instagram. I'm also open to emails, and I also do free Zoom calls. I might even have a connection in your area or someone I can suggest you reach out to whom I think would be a good match. I'd love to connect with you online, share more information about The Other's Day Brunch, or talk about what you can gain from joining Thrive After Infertility.

As you can see, there are plenty of options for reinvesting in your social life and discovering who you are and what you can be after infertility. Of course, opportunities change across localities, so there are probably some things I missed that you've thought of as a way to create connections with others in your area. Let's record those thoughts and any plans you want to put in place that might have come up for you while reading this chapter. Consider the following questions for your paper thinking today:

- What type of connection am I seeking? Athletic, intellectual, social, or otherwise?
- What are three places I could go to that would help connect me to others?
- When do I want to begin taking these actions?

16

Acknowledging Change in
Ongoing Relationships

Now that we've talked about how to handle icebreakers that revolve around children, let's address those long-standing relationships that might cause you discomfort now that you are on the other end of your infertility journey. You are not alone if you find yourself questioning your existing friendships, especially if there's a lot of mom and kid talk in your social gatherings. It can feel alienating to be the one person who can't contribute to the conversation. It can make you detach and disengage from the group and also compound feelings of alienation. It can be a real setback to all the work you've done on yourself to momentarily feel that you can't relate to your crew, your people, the girls who used to be your ride-or-dies.

Let me clarify that this chapter isn't encouraging you to sever ties because your friends have kids and you don't. It's simply meant to show that you matter in this equation, and you have options. You can always ask your friends ahead of time to not have completely kid-focused conversations, begin a one-on-one conversation with someone else to excuse yourself, and head to the bathroom if the group talk gets to be too much. And of course, you can always choose to sit out girls-night if it has become too much for you. But what if these approaches aren't enough or you're not finding the support you had hoped for among this group of longtime friends? That stings, and it can be a tough pill to swallow.

The truth is that people change, relationships take different paths, and people can outgrow one another. Think about all the things that have changed over the course of your life, from careers to hairstyles to hobbies. Friendships and social connections are no different. Old friends from childhood whom you may not see any longer aren't as close as they used to be. That work group you depended on for water cooler hang-outs and lunchtime conversation became less vital once you changed jobs. People change, circumstances change, your life has changed; there may be changes in your personal relationships as a result.

This is difficult for so many reasons. Because humans are social animals, it makes a lot of sense that we depend on our group for survival, connection, and support. When we feel someone slipping away, it can cause hurt feelings and even anxiety. As if the isolation you're already feeling through your infertility journey isn't enough, the thought of having one less option for a social partner might feel like it's compounding things. Sometimes it might be hard to judge if and when a friendship has run its course, but checking in with yourself is key. Are you getting together with this group or individual because you actually want to, or are you showing up because you're worried that you'll be judged if you don't? Connecting with your own needs first is important as you are emerging from your infertility journey, and those who truly care about you will understand that.

It's also important to remember that you may not have communicated your own needs to people, instead assuming they would automatically know how you would like to be handled or how certain situations should be treated. It might feel awkward or uncomfortable to open up the topic of a growing distance or friction within a friend group, but it's possible others aren't even aware of it or nobody wants to be the one to begin the conversation. As always, communication and trust are key.

I know that within my own friend groups, I took a lot of dips and turns in my involvement with them once I learned that my dream of being a mother would not be realized. My closest group of friends is quite the mix of motherhood statuses—there's a mom of identical IVF twins, a single mom, a foster mom, and me. They all found the motherhood that fit their path, while mine went a different route. There were times when it was hard to be around baby and family talk. There were times I judged myself and felt bad about my own character if I dragged my feet when it came time to make plans with them. I carried guilt when I didn't show up to their kids' birthday parties, visit their newborns, or send gifts upon the birth of their child. We have found other ways to connect as women and friends, even though I didn't always have the language to verbalize what I was going through, what I was burning for in our friendship during my darkest days through IVF. But with the fullest heart, I can say that we've found an amazing way to stay connected through all our unique journeys.

If you're not able to say the same about an individual or group of friends, it may be time to step back—not forever, maybe just as you're working through things and trying to sort out your needs. A lot of people judge themselves if they choose to complete a circle of friendship with someone. I have come to learn that people are intended to come in and out of our lives for certain reasons. It can be more damaging to force yourself to remain in a relationship if it is no longer serving you and that circle is ready to come to a close. Chemistry and connection can sputter out among friends just as they do in romantic relationships.

When you enter the part of your journey where you are ready to create new growth in your life and discover your meaning, some of your values may change. It's okay to ask yourself if you are no longer finding meaning or fulfillment in a particular relationship. It doesn't mean that the person themselves is not a valuable human being, it just means that your shared experiences may have come to an end. Your circle of friendship may have come to a completion; each of you has wonderful interests, experiences, and journeys that are growing in amazing ways, but in different forms.

It's important to remember that your friendship ending doesn't have to be dramatic and maybe doesn't even need to be directly addressed. There's no need to have a sit-down intervention, a wall of back-and-forth texts, or a dinner date that could end badly. People can easily drift apart, allowing the connection to fade in a natural and organic way. It's also very possible to maintain a relationship with this person but without the deeply intimate contact you had before. The relationship can take on a different form that may not be a friendship but can definitely be friendly. You can still carry affection for that person; it just shows up in a different way.

It may even be time to question the cornerstone of some friendships. There may be some connections you share that are based in an unhealthy bedrock. Perhaps you have a group you only engage with when you are partaking in buffering behaviors or one that is based on things that actually hold you back rather than help you grow and develop as a person. If there is a person or group of people that you are typically drinking, taking a smoke break, only talking shit, or gossiping or complaining with, it might be time to reevaluate your connection. Is your time together nourishing anymore? Or is it giving you permission to engage in some of your less desirable escapism habits?

One of the most important things to remember as you turn a spotlight onto your friendships and ask critical questions is that your story is not less valuable than anyone else's. Those conversations that other people can participate in when it turns to kids' birthday parties, the price of diapers, long nights with no sleep, and breastfeeding woes can feel very painful and make you feel as if you were an invisible cog in the group—the one that won't turn or grinds badly when these situations arise.

If you decide to maintain some of your relationships despite these circumstances, it's important to remember your own value and worth. No, you can't contribute to the kid conversation, and that's okay. Motherhood is part of their story, and you have your own life experiences that are just as relevant and important. You've fought your own battles and have emerged as a new woman, one who has found her purpose outside of motherhood. That story can't be taken from you, and it's as equally meaningful as anyone else's.

For your paper thinking today, I'd like you to consider some important questions when it comes to the status of some of your friendships that may feel like they are unraveling or have become less relevant to you.

- Why am I friends with this person?
- If I met this person today, would I still want to be friends with them?
- Why do I still have a connection with this person?
- Am I attracted to the idea of maintaining this friendship, or does the thought just make me feel tired and anxious?

These critical questions can help you determine why you are holding on to a friendship, and whether it is still serving you as you move forward on your journey to becoming the fulfilled, accomplished, and valued woman you are meant to be.

17

The Solution to the Drama

So far, we've talked a lot about how other people impact you, your feelings, and your environment. We've covered how to get comfortable with yourself and how to feel more in control when you are confronted with uncomfortable situations and conversational topics about your motherhood status. What you've been through is one of the most difficult things a woman can face, and you're ready to create a future that is fulfilling, purposeful, and full of successes. You deserve all of this. A life you adore is attainable and so within reach, but it doesn't just plop into your lap. So it's time for some tough love.

If you're anything like me, you've had days where everything was going great. You get up feeling positive and good about life and have a great day at work. On your way home you stop at the grocery store, you're in the produce section, and when you look up, who is in front of you? Susie Miller, a friend from high school you haven't seen in years. You want to run in the other direction because you know exactly how a catch-up conversation is going to go. And you're right—two minutes into the conversation, you've already been asked how many kids you have.

You are annoyed beyond belief that after all these years, this is where the conversation starts—not with your career, your husband, the nonprofit you started, or whatever it is you are most proud of in your life. When you use all your self-control to politely inform Susie that you weren't able to have children, she hits you with, "Stay positive, and it will happen!" Then she tells a story about her aunt's sister's cousin who got pregnant miraculously at the age of forty-five. You smile—because you're supposed to—and make it through the conversation. You bid her farewell and cringe your way through the hug and inevitable commentary that you should get together more often. By the time you make it back out to your car, the great day you were having has been blown to pieces, and you're mentally ripping Susie to shreds for being so invasive and intrusive.

I want to first acknowledge that feeling this way is normal. Of course it's a punch in the gut to have to dance around questions that still feel raw, but it is up to *you* to decide how you want to feel in these situations. What I have come to understand is that I was the problem.

I know that's a tough statement, but keep with me. When people would ask me any of the triggering family-related questions, it wasn't their words that put me into a tailspin, it was what *I* was thinking about *myself*. Susie wasn't standing there telling me that I was a failure as a woman because my body couldn't produce a child—*I* was telling myself that. It's easier for me to acknowledge now that I was the problem, and that's because I've found a solution!

We've talked a lot about how our brains are wired to keep us alive, and how anything that feels like a threat can automatically send us into a reactive state. We live in a modern world, but our brains are still primal, and when we have a strong reaction to something or someone, our brain identifies them as a threat and treats them as such. My brain wanted to tag someone like Susie as a danger to my well-being because my body went into a stress reaction around her—elevated heart rate, anxiousness, pulse quickening. These are signs of danger, and my brain decided that *Susie = Threat = Enemy*, when really Susie was just someone who could use some social skills and maybe some conversation coaching.

In short, our brains are drama queens. This is why they interpret everything so intensely, telling us on repeat that people are judging us, our childless life is pitiful, and we're going to die alone. It's a horrible cycle, but it's also your brain's job to keep you safe and help you prepare for triggering situations. Luckily for us, most people aren't judging us, life isn't terrible, and we're not going to die alone—but our brain wants us to be ready for that, just in case. And it is possible to control whether you hit the panic button every time your brain thinks you should.

So often we see other people as the source of our misery. They are assumptive, clueless with questions, and drain us of energy. But the truth is, it's not fully accurate that someone else can cause drama for you. What other people say and do are neutral circumstances; it's often the *thoughts you are having* about you that create those feelings and emotions. Other people's words and actions may be dramatic, but they do not have to cause drama. The drama comes as a response to your thoughts about what they've said or done. And yes, sometimes you may be triggered by comments or experiences; it still happens to me all these years into my childlessness, but it's less frequent and debilitating when I know that I can control my views of myself and my worthiness as an infertile woman without children.

If there is a friend group, a coworker, or a family member who you've labeled as someone who causes drama in your life, avoiding them is certainly an option, but you can also choose to learn how to manage your reactions so you can build emotional independence. Understanding that you can be in charge of the commentary in your brain about you, your infertility, and childlessness is going to become pure gold to you. When I learned this was possible, it changed my life, and I can't keep quiet about it. I want women to know that our self-perception in these situations is a beautiful option over teaching ourselves that avoidance is the answer.

When you decide someone else is toxic or overly dramatic, you're telling your brain that they are a problem in your life. Your brain listens and responds by treating any interaction with that person as a potential threat. This creates tension—your defenses go up, and even their harmless questions can feel like attacks. But here's the thing: The real issue isn't just the person or their behavior. It's how your mind is choosing to interpret the situation. The good news? You have the power to shift this. You don't have to give your emotional well-being away to others by labeling them as threats or obstacles. Instead, you can create boundaries that feel healthy without turning interactions into battlegrounds.

You might be bristling right now, thinking, *Oh, Lana, you've brought me so far and I've learned so much, and then boom! It turns out you're just like everyone else. You're judging me too and I'm closing this book now to go find someone who is actually supportive.* If you're feeling that way right now, it's okay! I totally get it, and I would have reacted similarly before I went through coaching and learned how to manage my own brain.

Let's reread that last paragraph, and really think about it. When we behave in a reactionary way, we are allowing someone else to exercise more control over our brain than ourselves. We've been accustomed to feel like a certain person can deem our worthiness, judge our situation, or prescribe what they think we should be doing. If you want less emotional drama in your life, stop believing that other people can cause it for you. They may think they're being supportive, but your brain interprets their words as personal judgments. It's time to ask if *your own thoughts* about your childlessness are toxic to you. Ironically, when I stopped labeling other people as the problem, I experienced the power that comes with managing my reactions. I want that emotional independence for you too.

Think about it like this: When you get a new appliance or piece of technology, it comes with an instruction manual. As humans we carry around our own instruction manuals for how people are supposed to act, what they should say and do so that we can remain happy, proud, and unaffected. It makes a lot of sense: We have expectations of others, and when they don't adhere to them, shit hits the fan, and we unravel because they didn't follow the instruction manual we had for them.

Let me be clear that this isn't the same as having personal boundaries. Having boundaries if you feel at risk of being emotionally, mentally, or physically harmed should be in place and always adhered to. But when someone like Susie in the produce aisle asks if you have kids or tells you to pray harder or that you should adopt, they don't realize that their comments aren't helpful. They didn't get the instruction manual of how to engage in conversation with you. Maybe this is the time to explain that you prefer not to discuss children or share your experiences with infertility. You can even gently suggest that such questions are not welcomed by all women. If this feels like a challenge, review the responses we covered in chapter 14 or refer to the list of responses on my website.

For your paper thinking, sit down and focus on one particular person in your life. It can be someone you have a great relationship with or someone who causes friction. If you were going to create an actual manual for how you would like them to interact with you, what would it say? Don't hold back; write down everything about how you would like this person to act toward you. Then, go through what you've written and ask yourself if some of those are worth sharing. Do these expectations seem realistic? What will you do or think about yourself if they are not met?

Likewise, you can even build an instruction manual for *yourself* rather than for others—a guidebook about how you want to feel in these sticky situations. It might include the story you tell yourself about the path you have been on and who you can become as a result of it. Remind yourself that you did all you were capable of and that your story isn't a tragedy that makes you a person to be pitied. Notice the feelings you have when you walk away from conversations, such as my fictional one with Susie, and come up with the antidote. Write it down so that you have a positive reference point when you find yourself reacting to an average conversation as if it were a threat.

Learning to train your brain is only part of the journey; having physical reminders that are tailored to your own experience will help you reach the confident, thriving future you!

18

The Distinction Between Addressing Your Needs and Being Selfish

What do you think of when you hear the word *selfish*? Probably nothing good. It brings to mind those who are self-centered and not empathetic, likely people you wouldn't enjoy spending time with. You might have even conjured an immediate picture of a person you know through work, a friend who has that character quirk, or even a family member who likely won't ever grow out of that particular mindset. I'm guessing one person that didn't come to mind was yourself—and I'm also guessing that you would never think of being selfish as a good thing. But guess what? It can be not only a positive aspect in your life when used appropriately but also a perfectly healthy one.

As women, a lot of us were raised to put others and their needs in front of our own, to do for others before we do for ourselves. And—to be clear—that is a beautiful way to live your life. When you offer yourself, moments of kindness, and gestures of goodwill to others, you are bringing joy and light to the world—but only if you do such things because you truly want to. When putting the needs of others before your own is happening at a rate that is a detriment to your own mental, social, and emotional health, it's time for you to consider focusing on yourself a little bit more and addressing what you need, want, and deserve.

To begin with, practicing self-care and recognizing your self-importance is not a form of narcissism. Focusing on yourself and knowing what your needs are is not a negative thing. It's nearly impossible to help and support others when you are depleted spiritually, emotionally, and physically. Acknowledging your own needs, knowing yourself, and understanding your own brain will put you in a place where you have so much more to contribute to the world in a way that genuinely feels good to both you and the person or group you are showing up for.

We're going to touch on an event that causes a lot of trepidation for women who are childless not by choice: invitations to kids' birthday parties. Prior to life coaching, when I would receive such an invitation, I didn't know how to say no. I knew I did not want to attend, but I also did not want the person inviting me to think I was so self-centered in my own grief that I couldn't celebrate their child. So I would attend out of a desire not to disappoint someone else, depleting my energy at a time when I was already struggling. The whole time I was there, pent-up disappointment and frustration built inside of me, but I perfected my Oscar-worthy performance that had people believing I was doing great and had emerged unscathed from fertility treatments that failed me. People would tell me how well I was doing and how strong I was. But I was lying—not only to them, but also to myself. I was taxing myself in ways that weren't necessary, just so I could appear to be unselfish and not self-centered.

Forcing yourself to do something like attend a first birthday party for your best friend's kid does no one any good—not you, not the host, not the other attendees. But you might go out of fear of judgment for yourself; because if you think you're a bad friend for not going, then most certainly other people will think that too. That well-trained brain of yours will let you wander into that place where you imagine you are the topic of conversation at the party—the friend who can't be happy for others because she's envious of their ability to have a baby.

It wasn't until I started acknowledging my need to preserve my emotional well-being that my nervous system calmed down. It needed a break from the act I was putting on day after day.

THE DISTINCTION BETWEEN ADDRESSING YOUR NEEDS AND BEING SELFISH

Not only at birthday parties, but also at work, church, and social functions. I didn't want to miss a beat because if I did, people would have an opportunity to judge me. I participated anyway, ignoring my needs and the fact that it's totally acceptable to take a step back from these overwhelming functions. This can be a hard thing for some of us to get our arms around; many of us are raised to believe that we should be doing and showing up for others. We are not supposed to struggle or show weakness, so we do what we've been taught. That may work in other parts of life, but when it comes to navigating childlessness after infertility, you're only going to inject more stress and emotional turmoil into your life.

You have a choice in this. If you are feeling constantly exhausted and like you never prioritize your own needs, wants, and desires, chances are you have not been practicing good self-care, and you are filling your time by putting the needs of others before your own. You can still be an amazing, giving, and loving person *and* put yourself first in situations where it is necessary. I can say this with authority because saying no to things I don't have the emotional bandwidth for is a practice I have adopted. I will never have children and I'm not going to raise a family; therefore, I treat myself with the love and compassion I would want to show to my children. If you can mother yourself and mother your life in the same way you would have your children's, you will create such a beautiful human within you. You'll give yourself the opportunity to explore what's important to you and what brings you joy because you're doing it for your own fulfillment versus doing it for someone else's when you think that's what they want you to do.

I can remember specific moments when I'd be driving to an

event that I just didn't have the space for emotionally or mentally and asking, *Why do I do this to myself?* I'm sure you've been there too, and it does not feel good. Not only are you going to show up inauthentically, but you're also diverting time and energy away from the things that you truly want to do, the things that will nourish you, help you grow, and contribute to your healing journey.

Your paper thinking is going to be a little more in-depth than usual, as breaking those learned bonds with the concept of being selfish is a difficult thing to do. I'd like for you to sit down with your calendar for the next month and take a hard look at it. Separate the things you are looking forward to from the ones that you are attending out of a sense of duty. Then, make a list of all the things you want to do this month, whether they are on the calendar or not.

Have you been meaning to get those seeds started for your garden but haven't had the chance yet? Is the fact that your car needs an oil change stressing you out, but there hasn't been time to take care of it? Have you set a weekly fitness goal that you haven't met, and it's making you feel bad about yourself? Is there a friend or family member whom you really want to catch up with, but you're feeling pressured to attend an extracurricular work event or accepted another invitation instead? List everything out, then ask yourself why these things are important to you and pay attention to your answers. Be honest with yourself and analyze what you are doing and why you are doing it. Are you participating in things or attending events because you want to or because someone else wants you to, and you're afraid of disappointing them?

Now, commit to being "selfish" for just one month and see if you can build a new relationship with being selfish! Through this exercise, you will get a better understanding of what fills your schedule and why—and if it's nourishing you or depleting you. When you devote yourself to things, places, and people that aren't fulfilling you, it empties your gas tank to where you don't have anything left for yourself or for the people in your life whom you want to connect with more fully. You'll get to a point where you'll actually enjoy doing things because you genuinely want to do them for yourself, which in turn results in you partaking in activities that you want to be a part of—which means someone else is getting joy out of your genuine involvement as well. When you show up from the sheer love in your heart, you are going to realize how much lighter it is to show up for yourself and the people around you.

19

You Can Always Adopt! And Other Clueless Things People Say

There are so many things that can cause discomfort for women who are childless not by choice. Sometimes just walking down the sidewalk can be a minefield, and navigating Target around Mother's Day or during back-to-school season can feel like an unfair reminder of things we miss out on. We've talked about options for handling feelings of disappointment these occasions often stir up, but what about handling comments and suggestions from other people? We've already discussed how social gatherings and meeting new people can be difficult at times and how interactions with old friends or family members may feel invasive. While we are all unique individuals with our own stories, I've noticed some common themes my coaching clients are often confronted with.

One of the hardest things I navigated when my IVF journey ended without a child was people feeling sorry for me. Having someone say, "I'm so sorry," when I explained why I didn't have kids was difficult for me. It made me feel like the life I was living was pitiful. Like I was the worst-case scenario. Up until my diagnosis of unexplained infertility, I saw myself as successful—a total achiever. So it felt belittling to be someone who was pitied. The repetition of being told how sorry everyone else was that I couldn't get pregnant grated on my nerves. It felt like my life was worthy of a sympathy card every single day, which was simply not the case. But even worse were the comments people with kids would say when I told them I couldn't have one.

"Lucky you! You can have my kids anytime; just ask!" was a disturbingly common response when I shared I was unable to have children. Others chimed in with remarks like, "Kids aren't all they're cracked up to be" and "I'd kill to have all that free time!" I'm sure they didn't realize how deeply hurtful such flippant comments were, especially about something I'd dreamed of for my entire life. Those words were hard to hear, and interactions like that could send me into a spiral.

I've spent a lot of time deciding how I want to handle other people's comments, and I strive to help my clients develop a different perspective when they encounter painful situations like these. I've come to realize that it had nothing to do with what people said and everything to do with what I was making their words mean about me and my childlessness.

I truly believe people who express sympathy are genuine in their statement, and they mean to show support by their words. They don't know how hard the words *I'm sorry* hit me. Ultimately, I learned that it wasn't their statements that were causing my annoyance, but my own internal reaction to them. Pity isn't comfortable to me, and I didn't like believing I was the target for their sympathy. My reaction was based on my own beliefs and fears, rooted in a place deep down inside that was going to need a lot of work.

The flippant responses about farming out their own kids or the bold statements that being a mom isn't all that great anyway are no different. I can't control what other people say to me, and as much as I wish I could, I can't always control the environment around me. What I can control is my reaction to their words and the story I tell myself about who I am because of my infertility. Like you, I've got my own particular thorn that sticks in my side, a topic that inevitably surrounds the topic of infertility: adoption. I'm sure you've heard this immediate rejoinder to your statement that you can't conceive: "But you can always adopt!" People who say this don't know about the years of conversations, the treatments, the hours spent in waiting rooms, long phone calls with doctors and fertility clinics where every possible avenue was explored.

But there's a deeper thrust here, one I feel every time the topic comes up. Yes, I can always adopt. I know this. Here's the truth: I have decided not to. There are a lot of reasons for this, but when I share this with someone, I am making myself vulnerable to their judgment. I fully believe that my husband and I made the right decision for us when we chose not to adopt. However, there have been times when I have felt an unspoken implication that I must not have wanted a baby that badly since I didn't exhaust all options. It often feels as if people think of my decision not to adopt is a selfish one—that I deprived a deserving child of a home.

The decision to adopt—or not to adopt—is a complicated one. So many unknowns surround this option, from prenatal care to genetic or family-related health issues. The fear of heartbreak. After years of being on the infertility roller coaster, I was not sure I could put myself through the emotional turmoil that surrounds adoption. Just like pregnancy, there are no guarantees that you will be able to take a child home if you go the adoption route. Even if you do make it through all the hurdles to be deemed an acceptable adoptive parent and have identified the baby or child you are hoping you can call your own, the birth parents may change their mind about giving up the child or want their parental rights back.

I suffered too many disappointments to knowingly open myself up to more. That is what really drove my decision not to adopt. If you're like me, you may have been in situations before where you've had to defend that decision or felt like you were supposed to apologize for it. I'm here to tell you that is not the case. Adoption is a beautiful choice for some, and I have a very close friend who has found great joy and meaning in it. But, it was not the choice for us.

For your paper thinking today, I'd like you to consider what feelings come up for you when you are in situations like these. Ask yourself the following questions:

- What comes up for me when someone comments flippantly?
- What am I thinking about me?
- How does that thought feel?

20

Will My Marriage Be Enough?

This book is full of content that may be new to you, and it may be strange to think you have as much control of how you feel as you do. This chapter might set you back on your heels because the emotions you'll encounter when you dive into this topic are a little different. All along, we've been talking about being childless not by choice and how to navigate the world without something you always hoped you would have. Now though, I'd like to talk about something that may be equally complex—the thought of losing something that you do have.

Many of my clients tell me that when they find out they can't have children, they consider the person next to them, their spouse or partner, the man they chose to spend their lives with and who they thoughtfully considered as the person who would father their children. An uncomfortable thought that often occurs after becoming childless is: *Will my marriage be enough? Is the bond I have with this person going to be enough to fulfill a life if it's just the two of us when we both assumed there would be children present?*

There are so many complicated feelings—guilt being a major one—that arise when you discover you can't have children. When you are the one with the infertility diagnosis, you may feel as if you have let your partner down by not being able to conceive, and by extension, maybe your parents or your in-laws who are missing out on the opportunity to be grandparents. Now your partner is left with the harsh reality that their decision to be with you means their own dream of parenthood is gone. The terrible f-word, *failure*, can raise its head again, and your internal friction of dealing with the negative thoughts you're having about yourself can become external, causing fights and rifts within the relationship.

Many of us choose our partner with the idea of future children in mind. You look at a person and think about their qualities and attributes and wonder what those would be like combined with your own. You daydream about whether your children would look more like him or you, and when you watched them interact with small children or babies, your heart melted as you dreamed about the day that tenderness would be directed at a child that you created together. When all those possibilities are taken from you, you're left with the reality that it's going to be the two of you for the rest of your lives—and no matter how strong your bond is, that can be really scary, and even make you wonder if your partnership will become a lonely one or can stand the test of time. Questioning the strength of your bond may bring up thoughts of self-judgment. You feel deceitful that you are having these second thoughts about someone who's been by your side through so much. I assure you, you are not the only one who's been here.

I struggled with these problems in my marriage as well. A child can be a buffer in a relationship, something that you both can funnel your love and affection into even if things might be rocky at the moment. A child will be a shared, common interest for the rest of your lives, a permanent bond that can also be a bridge between you when the waters get a little rough. Through my life coaching, I chose to do the hard work of examining this question, and I discovered that I have a beautiful opportunity to spend the rest of my life with someone I love—a person I call my husband. And my desire to prioritize that made such a difference for me!

On our thirteenth anniversary, I decided that Jack and I should have a long talk about what goals we have as a couple.

I wanted to really dig deep and mutually decide what we want to do more of as a couple and what we want to do less of in our relationship. Notice how I phrased that—doing more of something or less of something doesn't mean that you're starting from zero or stopping something entirely. The idea that your spouse may want less of something in your relationship can be frightening. It can feel like you're doing something wrong, that he would prefer to do a certain activity with friends rather than you, or maybe he even would like to be alone more often because you're not an enjoyable person to be with. That is absolutely not the case, and it's not a problem only childless couples deal with. While your union is truly a coming together, you have to remember that a partnership takes two people, and both of those people are individuals who have their own needs, friendships, and activities outside of the relationship.

Jack and I love to hike together. It's a big part of our lives, a shared hobby that we both enjoy. On a recent trip to California, we explored the Redwood forests. It was so quiet, so peaceful, and it was just the two of us on the path—there wasn't even another car in the parking lot. There was a huge comfort for me in the fact that we could be together in that solitary place, and I felt completely fulfilled and safe. So safe, in fact, that I felt comfortable sharing with him that I once questioned whether our marriage would be enough. I had never shared that with him before, and I told him that one of the things I'd had the privilege of helping my clients work through is whether a union between two people is enough without children.

He was an honest and open listener and never made me feel like I was a bad person, that I hadn't loved him or believed in our marriage enough. We shared a beautiful embrace under the

Redwoods, and I told him that I knew he and I were enough. I know that our love is enough. I know there are other things outside of parenthood that we're going to grow and do together, and also some separations will occur as each of us grows as individuals and finds fulfillment in small ways outside of the marriage.

Jack and I are both very independent people, which is a benefit in our relationship and in our individual lives. But when I found myself questioning if my marriage was going to be enough, it felt shameful. It felt like I was questioning something I'd never had doubts about before, but I was left holding the bag when we found ourselves childless. It was devastating. Before I had the courage to share these thoughts with my husband, it felt like I was being inauthentic in the relationship, which led to a feeling of disconnection. There was a deep fear I now realize was actually quite simple. I was asking myself, *What if we run out of things to do?*

Our lives were supposed to be full of diaper changes and homework, soccer practice and swimming lessons. We were supposed to be stretched thin, overtaxed, exhausted, and worn out—and deep down loving every second of it. I remember early on after our fertility journey ended, one of my biggest worries was literally running out of things to talk about with Jack. We would sit at dinner and have the conventional "how was your day" conversation where each of us shared about our day at work, what we were going to have for dinner the next day, or what we thought we might do that weekend. And honestly, it all felt very unexciting. It made me question whether we had what it would take to feel fulfilled and connected to one another without having a child to share.

Navigating this question in your mind is difficult, and one of the ways I worked my way through it was by remembering what it was that had attracted me to Jack in the first place. I asked myself what it was that made me want to say yes to spending the rest of my life with him and creating a union together. And of course the possibility of children was part of that, but there were so many other things that weren't related to parenting or motherhood—and those things are of great value. They are worth spending a lifetime experiencing. Understand that there are going to be many challenges in your future, but knowing that there's someone by your side who loves you even if you aren't going to be parents together, that they have chosen to stick with you and stay with you is a blessing, and it is one you are deserving of.

For your paper thinking today, I'd like for you to write down the things that are going well or working well in your partnership. Then list all the things you'd like to do more of as a couple, and maybe some things you want to do less of as well. Maybe you'd like to watch less Netflix and take more walks after dinner. Maybe you want more hobbies you can explore together or vice versa—perhaps you'd like more independent time to experience some things on your own. There are so many possible combinations of things that you want more or less of, activities for you to experience together or on your own. Let your mind wander and remember it's never too late to discover your meaning—or the meaning of your marriage!

21

Telling Your Story and Educating Others

There are so many aspects of everyday life that can be unexpectedly stressful for women with infertility, and one of the most triggering for some is the OB/GYN annual exam. Many of us dread our yearly PAP, and most don't think twice about what comes before putting your feet in the stirrups: the routine paperwork and general health questions, sitting in a waiting room packed with expectant moms. Returning to the same office where you went for monitoring, blood draws, and maybe even retrievals and implantations can feel incredibly triggering.

At a recent annual exam, I answered the first few intake questions easily enough—height and weight—but when I was asked the date of my last period I hesitated, and not because I didn't know the answer. It was 1,627 days ago. Does that seem really specific? I could say this with certainty because I still have the ovulation app on my phone I once used to monitor my menstrual cycles. That's more than four years—years that marked a time of my coming to terms with the fact that I would never be a mother. But there was more. Next, they asked if I was still on birth control, how many pregnancies I'd had, and if I had any children. In the past, I'd always put my head down and shouldered the pain, answering the questions simply to move forward with the exam.

This time, I didn't. This time, I asked my own questions.

The medical assistant was very sweet and kind, so I was careful to pose my thoughts in a nonaggressive way, as she was only doing her job and checking the boxes on the computer she was being asked to check. But I'd been coming to the same doctor for some time, and in fact, I had been a patient in this office during my fertility treatments. I felt as if the information I was being asked to regurgitate each year should be available in my chart without having to put me through the emotional strain of telling someone yet again, "No, I don't have any children."

When the doctor entered the exam room, I explained that these seemingly benign intake questions can actually be very difficult for those of us who have been through the gauntlet of infertility, and that they might consider becoming more accommodating. Perhaps they could flag charts or profiles ahead of time so that the office staff can access the patient's medical records with the information already filled in. This would save the patient the painful experience they will have to relive again next year, even though the answers will remain the same. I discussed this with the doctor to build some more awareness around this topic within their office.

My OB/GYN was very receptive to the idea and apologized if I'd been made uncomfortable. I told her that I'd done a lot of work on myself and have come to a place where I am able to navigate questions and also find the courage to speak up for others in my community who might not be able to manage this situation as easily. I made my doctor familiar with the work I do as a life coach and the impact I am making as an infertility advocate. She not only listened to what I had to say but also acknowledged that there had to be a way to prepare for patients like me so as not put them through the cookie cutter questions that other women might breeze through easily. She even asked me for resources I could offer that might help the office do a better job for women like us.

I walked out of the appointment feeling something that I hadn't felt when leaving an OB/GYN before—pride and a sense of ownership over my journey. I hadn't silenced myself for fear of rocking the boat or being judged; I'd spoken up and taken a stance by explaining that for some of us, it's not simple at all. I'd spoken up not only for myself but also for you, and for all of the women out there like us, who might not be in a place where they have been able to find their voice yet.

If you're at a place where you are ready, join me. It only takes one or two women pushing back against the status quo to change the intake process for you and the women behind you who don't have the words yet to speak up. Childless women should be spared these invasive questions, but also be provided with resources to help them deal with their unexpected childlessness.

Infertility needs and deserves education, and not just in the offices of medical practitioners. When I think about the little girl I was, watching the women around me become mothers, I simply assumed that my life would follow the same path. I would get married and become a mother while also working and balancing other life obligations. But always, the center of my perceived future purpose came through motherhood. Now, though, I hope that women like you and I can be present and visible in the lives of young girls so they will be able to see that happiness and a purposeful life for a woman doesn't necessarily always include children. Even if *speaking up* doesn't necessarily fit where you are right now, simply *showing up* as an example of a thriving woman can help shape the perceptions of young people.

If you're more comfortable and would like to consider sharing your story, think about younger women in your life who might need some basic education about fertility if they want to meet their personal, social, and career goals. When I got married at thirty-five, I never dreamed I'd have trouble getting pregnant—especially because I always had a regular cycle. I simply assumed that getting pregnant would fall into the natural line of things. I wasn't expecting to receive a medical diagnosis of unexplained infertility. No one prepared me for the possibility of seeing a specialist in order to get pregnant, and I certainly wasn't aware of acronyms like IUI and IVF and that egg freezing may have been an option to consider in my younger years. Not knowing about some processes is one thing, but I have learned that many young women aren't well informed about even the most common ones. My guest appearances on podcasts and national news have taught me that many young women are ill informed and lack awareness around advanced maternal age.

Also, there is so much to be gained by talking to policy and lawmakers about the lack of reliable and available healthcare that covers IVF. States need to understand that women deserve the option of motherhood; it is not a privilege, it is a right for us to have access to appropriate care. Treatment should not be available only to those who can afford it or have healthcare plans inclusive of fertility treatments. Friends of mine in foreign countries are offered reproductive treatments as part of their benefits of being a citizen, while I ended up paying, at an extraordinary expense, for a private healthcare plan simply to cover my IVF treatments.

Finally, it's important that employers be aware of what women in our position need. A doctor's appointment may be scheduled at the last minute for a retrieval or implantation. Medications that must be taken on a strict schedule may mean that we need to carve out time during our workday to adhere to our protocols. Often overlooked is the delicate aftermath that accompanies a pregnancy loss. I know many women who have experienced pregnancy loss only to be expected to show up at work the next day. Little to no concern was given to their emotional state.

There are so many important reasons to tell your story—when you are ready—to all kinds of people. In the workplace, among family members and friends, and even in the halls of government. Our stories matter and can never be heard if they are not told. You are moving into your future as a strong, fulfilled woman who can serve as a beacon of light to others who may walk the same path. Whether you choose to speak or lead by example, know that you have an impact on everyone around you, and that there is an entire community behind you, supporting you and loving you along the way!

Your Relationship with Holidays and Events

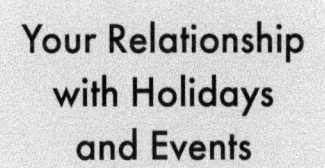

PART 3

22

Happy Holidays . . . Maybe?

There are regular days that can be stressful for those of us who are childless not by choice. From coworkers making pregnancy announcements to the invasive questions at social gatherings, it can feel like every twenty-four-hour cycle contains triggering moments. Then there are those special days on the calendar, the holidays that we come together to celebrate. We humans are social animals, and we have cultural dates and milestone markers that mean something to us collectively as well as individually. For us childless women, sometimes the holidays feel like a pressure cooker containing all the necessary ingredients to make you spiral: your personal disappointments, unfulfilled expectations in regard to what you dreamed these holidays would be like as a parent, and memories of your own childhood holidays, now bittersweet as you believe that you won't be able to enjoy holidays any longer.

To begin with, I'd like to acknowledge that it's okay to be sad around the holidays. It's a time of nostalgia for many—not just for women who are childless. But many people carry an expectation that you should be joyous and celebratory during the holidays, and for women who are childless or are navigating infertility, the pain can be all the more pronounced. If you're not feeling as festive as you had hoped—or as others expect you to be—remember that over time this is manageable and modifiable. It will just take a little bit of awareness on your part. So, by first giving ourselves permission to be sad, we are acknowledging that there is a void attached to the holidays for us, and that is okay. What you *think about yourself* for not being in love with the holidays is what will make the difference in your life, which comes back to your thoughts affecting your emotions.

You may feel melancholy around some holidays. You likely had expectations for what Christmas mornings would look like or treasure fond memories of coloring Easter eggs when you were a child. A lot of your dreams for your future may have revolved around expanding those memories with your own children. But now that you know that won't be a possibility, holidays in general can feel empty. So where do we go from here? This is the key to leading yourself out of a place of living in your past, so you can start to move forward and create abundance in your future.

As we grow older, things change in our lives. Friends relocate, family members pass away. Life is fluid and constantly changing, which means that the holidays of our past can never be fully duplicated. When you tell yourself that things need to remain the same to be fulfilling, you sell yourself—and the holidays themselves—short.

You have the amazing power to choose the thoughts you want to have so you can create the future you desire. Regardless of what celebrations used to be like, you can move forward into this year's celebration with love in your heart for the way you felt before; but also with the joy of discovering something new. You can also choose to think differently about the holidays you want to have. You can create whatever it is that you want.

Thanksgiving is often viewed as the kickoff to the holiday season. Recently, I was working with a client who shared with me her dread of participating in her family tradition of each person at the table saying what they are thankful for in their lives. She has a supportive husband and is successful in her career, but she is unable to get pregnant. It had been her goal for so long that it made the other achievements in her life pale in comparison. In our session, we talked about whether it's possible to be thankful for a life without motherhood. And the answer that we landed on was, "Heck, yes!"

You have a wonderful opportunity to attach new meaning to each holiday in your life. I used to wake up on Christmas mornings and feel like it was just another mile-marker along the path of infertility, another year without a child to open presents with. But once I started noticing my thoughts and how they were creating my feelings, I discovered I could create new Christmas traditions, and that made all the difference. I have the amazing and beautiful blessing of waking up next to a man I love every day. On Christmas mornings, we've created opportunities to celebrate our love and relationship. No year is exactly the same—sometimes it's through a beautifully written note, gift giving, having breakfast together, hosting a family celebration for our extended family, or just enjoying a day without work, a day where we can be a couple moving through the world together.

So many of us have amazing success stories that we don't even give ourselves credit for. The lack of gratitude we offer ourselves can hold us back from creating a future of abundance and from viewing the present holidays as nothing more than a social slog that only brings up feelings of sadness. Many of us avoid giving ourselves credit because we've somehow decided that it's boastful or egotistical to point out what's wonderful about us.

I'm here to remind you that you are worth celebrating. There's so much greatness in your life. And there's no need to judge yourself if it's been a while since you've acknowledged it. You should commend yourself for wanting to get on the other side of this feeling of emptiness, even if it still feels like a stretch.

Recognize the courage it takes to do the work you are doing. Not everyone has the vision that you do and the desire to create a life they love—even when it turned out so differently than expected. But you do, and that alone is the launching point to creating it.

This topic is so nuanced that I created the "Learn to Love Your Life After Failed IVF So You Can Start to Thrive Again" guide to help you navigate some of the complexities you might be experiencing. You can download it for free at lanamanikowski.com/holiday. In it, you'll find journaling prompts that will help you sort through the mixed bag of emotions you may be feeling during holiday celebrations, with a few affirmations sprinkled in to help remind you of how magnificently wonderful you are.

As you've come to learn, the thoughts you have directly correlate to the way you are feeling, and the guide is designed to help you get a better understanding of how your thoughts around the holiday season are making you feel. When you learn how to speak and think of your life in a way that gives you power and intention, you'll be amazed by the control you can have. The affirmations I offer in the guide are a launching point to help you connect to feelings of self-worth. The journal prompts will help you to see that creating new traditions, celebrating holidays in a different way, and feeling meaningful around the holidays really is possible; you just have to give yourself the opportunity to decide what that might look like without children and that you are worth an abundant future.

Not having a child does not sentence you to a life of annual holidays that seem empty and not worth celebrating. Coming up in this section we'll spend time thinking about specific holidays, as well as certain times of the year, in detail.

For your paper thinking, I'd like you to look at your life from an outsider's perspective. When you have a conversation with someone or people are curious about you, imagine that any discussion of motherhood is off the table. What would you talk about? What are three things about you that you think are interesting? What are you proud of in your life?

Hold on to your answers every day of your life, not just holidays! And remember, it's never too late to discover your meaning—or to create new meaning around holidays.

23

Halloween and Christmas

You typically don't see Halloween and Christmas mentioned in the same breath, but those of us who are childless not by choice can pinpoint exactly what these two holidays have in common—they are both very kid-centric. From the well-meaning weatherman who uses radar to track Santa's sled on Christmas Eve to the lines of costumed children out trick-or-treating, these two holidays in particular can have a very heavy impact on the emotions of a woman without children. The holiday blues can seem inevitable, but the truth is they are *optional*. It may not seem easy now, but you can learn to be more connected to how you feel. Learning that skill has offered me the greatest amount of freedom, confidence, and purpose.

That doesn't mean the holidays might not feel overwhelming at times! From the endless and unavoidable ads featuring happy families to the dreaded family events and social gatherings, it can feel like every turn in your day might include a steel trap just waiting for you to step on it. Being childless isn't the only element that can take you by surprise. When I was going through IVF, I had put on quite a bit of weight—and we all have that one family member who likes to point out who looks different than they did last year at Christmas dinner. In short, some days it seems like everywhere you go, the world is waiting to remind you of what you don't have. So, of course, you are going to have some not-so-wonderful emotions surrounding certain holidays—and that's okay.

There is a sensationalized expectation in our society that everyone should be happy, particularly around Christmas. For many people—not just those without children—the "most wonderful time of the year" can feel like the exact opposite. We create so much anxiety for ourselves because in our hearts we are not feeling the way we think we should be. For me, that word came up a lot: *should*. And that big, bad word can show up at any holiday, or really any day at all.

I should have kids to sit on Santa's lap. I should have a child to shop for Halloween costumes with. I should be stronger. I should be happy just like everyone else. I should be smiling at Christmas dinner. I should be able to get through the back-to-school aisle without crying. I should not get so angry when Aunt Sally asks me about my ticking biological clock or Uncle Henry comments that it looks like I've been eating for two.

But here's a question, and it's one we haven't even asked ourselves. Is that how we want to feel? Is that truly how we feel in our hearts? Suddenly, we flip a page on a calendar, and our feelings turn into a snow globe of magic and joy or bite-size candy bars and pumpkin-shaped buckets? Of course not, and it's an unfair expectation we feel society has put on us. When we create anxiety for ourselves because we're not feeling a certain way, we're telling ourselves that there is something fundamentally wrong with ourselves. We buy in to this old, created story that actually negates our ability to enjoy life where we are right now.

When you tell yourself a story of how any holiday *should* be, it confines you. Your brain—that old frenemy—gets overloaded and is constantly looking for opportunities to point out when you aren't experiencing an event in the way you think you should. When you do this, it gives focus to the parts of your life that feel lacking, and the negatives begin to compound. But take a second and consider this statement: You have already survived 100 percent of your worst days. You are here, you are whole, and you are allowed to enjoy the parts of your life that feel good. The holidays can give you a great opportunity to show up as the person you are today and recognize the new potential of what holidays can mean for you.

You are a strong, powerful, resilient woman who shows up every day because you've got the courage to keep going. This is the story you need to tell yourself; it's a true story and one that you can absolutely believe in when you are about to walk into a holiday dinner, drive down the street on trick-or-treat night, or enter any other situation where you think people may feel sorry for you. Yes, you wish you could have had a child and your family wishes that for you too. But instead of adopting this story of melancholy that makes you feel weak, remind yourself that you are not lacking as a woman or are a less valuable member of your family, community, or society in general.

What if this actually means you are the strong one? What if someone around that dining room table, or navigating the crowded crosswalk, admires you because they know what you went through, and they are in awe of how you show up. Despite what you have been through, you are somebody who is still so strong and powerful. When you learn how to navigate the story not of how your holidays *should* be but rather how you *want* them to be, this is where your power comes from.

You have an old story inside your head, the one where you had a child and you had the opportunity to share all the holiday traditions and experiences of your own childhood with them. But when you create a new story in your mind and stay firm with it, you can determine how you want your holidays to be, and that might not include the activities, celebrations, and rituals that seem to be rinse-and-repeat every year within your family. What if you decide with your partner that you are creating your own tradition that doesn't have to be in accordance with the way that things have been done for fifty years in your family?

There is a new version of you, and you can show up as her, knowing that you are just as amazing as everyone else in that room because that's who you believe you are. You don't have to show up and absorb the sadness that other people might feel for you or apologize for the fact that you don't have a big family in tow. You don't have to be a person who is sad during the holidays—or really at any point in the calendar year. You can be somebody who's at peace and powerful and meaningful in the human body and the human existence you have today.

You do not have to celebrate in a way that you think you *should* be celebrating or in the way that other people believe you *should*. You can celebrate how you *want* to. There is so much more growth opportunity and a sense of lightness when you show up being who you want to be instead of who others think you should be. Align yourself with what you value and what you want to have, because grief doesn't have to define your holidays—any of them.

Define your holidays by taking an inventory of what's important to you and finding something meaningful that might help you reinvent the story of what a certain date means. Maybe you have a cousin you only see at Christmas and reconnecting with them can be a great motivation to enjoy the holiday dinner. Maybe there's a great Halloween-themed dessert or food you've always thought was clever or cute; your contribution to the party every year can be creating this tradition of your now-famous marshmallow pie. The possibilities and combinations of your unique, amazing self are available to you every day, and you have the power within you to create a new story about what holidays mean for you.

For your paper thinking, I'd like you to think about a few things that make you proud, whether it's your work performance, a particular skill, or the relationship you have with a friend or your spouse. Make a list of some of your strongest attributes and revisit it when you know a triggering holiday or calendar date is coming up so that you can remind yourself of all the amazing gifts you have to offer the world, even if they might not fit the mold of what the world is expecting right now. Likewise, think about some of the holidays that have been difficult for you in the past and consider how you can bring your talents and gifts to the table to create new traditions for yourself—and maybe even everyone else—so that you can reclaim that day on the calendar and redefine it for the strong, powerful woman that you are.

24

Mother's Day

For years, every May brought with it a sense of dread. So many emotions would come up for me during this month—the one that holds the most triggering holiday of all, Mother's Day. I would always feel such a jolt around this time because the messaging, advertisements, and celebration that surround this date are so pervasive. Grocery stores have grab-and-go bouquets at the front entrance. Billboards everywhere tout the importance of mothers in everyone's lives. Restaurants offer specials and remind you to make your reservations to honor your grandmother, mother, wife, sister, or daughter. And let's not even get started on trying to shop the greeting card aisle in Target for anything *other* than that. I'm sure you—and every other childless woman out there—has had similar experiences, and it's no wonder a date that's made up on a calendar can cause so much to come up for us and trigger feelings of loneliness that make us question our relevance as women.

So let's talk about why this peculiar date has such an impact on us. I'd like to start by saying that it's okay to feel sadness around Mother's Day. First, we need to acknowledge that, as much as we'd like, the world doesn't revolve around us and our feelings this weekend. People have every right to enjoy and celebrate this event with their own mothers, daughters, sons, and significant others. Mother's Day doesn't have to feel like a personal affront if you're able to step back from your knee-jerk, emotional reactions—which are totally understandable—and recognize that, while it may carry some difficult feelings for you, others are interacting with it in their own way as well.

Just like other holidays, there can be a social expectation when it comes to your emotional setting, and I'm here to let you know that there is nothing wrong with you if your inner thoughts and feelings don't automatically conform with everyone else's. Why would they? You are an individual person, with a different path from theirs, living out a life story that has its own beginning, middle, and end. There is no right way to feel about this or any other day, so let's acknowledge that your feelings are exactly that: yours.

It's so common for my clients to tell me they feel embarrassment, shame, or even depleted when it comes to this holiday. Recently, I was working with a client who told me she feels very selfish around Mother's Day because as an adult, she has only associated it with her own feelings and a sense of emptiness. She felt like she had forgotten the bigger picture and wasn't celebrating her own mother as a result of her negative thoughts. The heaviness she carried inside about this important holiday made it difficult for her to genuinely celebrate the love, affection, and gratitude she feels for her own mother, which made her feel as if she had made the date all about herself without taking others into consideration. I'm sure that's something many of us can relate to.

Mother's Day carries a particular significance for me as my birthday is May 14, and the two typically fall close together—sometimes the very same day—on the calendar. We'll talk about how our own birthdays impact our childlessness in another chapter, but ultimately the same tools have helped me navigate both situations. I allow myself the grace to recognize what I need and not judge myself for it. Judging yourself for the emotions you are having simply compounds them. I personally treat Mother's Day as an opportunity to show up for my mom while also recognizing my own needs.

I've hosted a Mother's Day brunch at my house every year for my mom, sister, and beloved mother-in-law (who is sadly now deceased). It has become a tradition they all look forward to, as do I. The entertaining, preparing food, and filling my house with guests keeps me busy and creates a new tradition that allows all of us to celebrate motherhood, sisterhood, and family, without me having to focus on my inability to have a child. I've made an agreement with myself to honor what I need for me so I can be emotionally present the best way I can. It's a win-win for all of us. I don't have to let my own sadness overshadow the love and gratitude that I feel in my heart for my own mother and extended family.

It took a while for me to arrive at this place. As I navigated my journey through infertility, I really had to pull myself together to even be present on Mother's Day. I felt judgment for myself as I stood in the card aisle, trying to pick out a card that honored this wonderful, amazing woman in my life—but really I was only focused on my own thoughts and feelings at the moment. That judgment combined with what I perceived as a failure in my own childlessness created a situation where I really had to muster up a lot of energy to feel any desire to celebrate my mom and how she helped shape much of who I am today.

If you recognize a yearning to support yourself, please do not judge yourself. You are not alone. You are not a bad person. You are not selfish for feeling sadness around a day that you dreamed of celebrating with your own children. It only makes sense that this might be a sad day for you, when you had the expectation of being a mom and had that experience taken away from you. It's not only understandable but normal for you to feel a little bit empty around Mother's Day.

So many of us have feelings of resentment associated with

Mother's Day. Maybe your best friend's social media post about her kids making her breakfast in bed brought up some envy. Maybe the mom-and-daughter spa day your sister had—complete with matching mani-pedi pics that were shared in a family group chat—caused a sense of disconnection for you. Maybe the coworker who shared her newly discovered pregnancy right before the weekend made you feel bad not only about *this* year's holiday, but now you're dreading *next* year's as well, when she'll be celebrating something that you wanted so badly and don't get to participate in.

Make no mistake about it—this time of year is hard. So many times the phrase that popped up in my mind over and over during the month of May felt so childish, so simple, but yet so true: *It doesn't seem fair.* It doesn't seem fair that my best friend got pregnant so easily without really trying. That I invested so much time, money, and emotion into this singular goal and was still cheated of motherhood. It can feel childish and silly when these emotions arise, but it's important to show yourself compassion and remember you are allowed to have these feelings—in fact, it makes sense for you to feel this way!

The truth is that it may never feel good when Mother's Day comes around. Even with all the work I do—and am continuously doing—on myself, that holiday always causes a little twinge in my heart. There is nothing wrong with me for feeling this way; I am not broken—and neither are you. Regardless of what emotion you're feeling around Mother's Day, remember to feel it without judging yourself. Then, ask yourself what you can do to take that compassion a step further. Do something for yourself or find something or someone to celebrate. Maybe you can be in charge of the Mother's Day celebration in your family or, if your mom isn't local or if she isn't with us anymore, call a friend and ask if it would be okay for you to join their family for the weekend. Are there other women in your world who don't have kids or don't have their kids nearby? Give them a buzz. Find something to do together.

If you find comfort in solitude, practice some self-care by preparing a plan for your Mother's Day weekend. Make yourself your favorite meal or indulge in a dessert that you only allow yourself on special occasions. Create a playlist of your favorite movies and get comfortable on the couch if that is what will bring you some contentment this Mother's Day.

Perhaps reaching out and offering comfort to others is something you find fulfilling. If that's the case, find a local soup kitchen and ask if they are looking for help on Mother's Day. Contact a women's shelter and see if there's something you can do for them, especially considering some of these women may be separated from their children. Buy up all those bouquets that made you feel so bad at the grocery store and drop them off at a nursing home, asking the staff to deliver them to the residents who might need their own pick-me-up on that important day or whose children are unable to come see them. There are so many ways you can create connections with others!

My desire to feel connected around Mother's Day has resulted in a major development in my life, and it's one of the things that I am most proud of: I created the annual Other's Day Brunch. I love connecting with others and also drawing connections between other people. So I decided to host an event that's open to anyone feeling a lot of emotion around Mother's Day. The brunch is about bringing together women who are seeking connection at a time that has historically been difficult or challenging for them. It's about celebrating their contributions to this world and everything they do every day when they show up as the proud, independent, beautiful women they are. Maybe they aren't moms, maybe they're missing their own moms, or maybe their own children aren't able to be with them on that day. Really, it's for anyone who feels like an *other* on Mother's Day!

The Other's Day Brunch was designed to create community with other women who relate to your story and want to reclaim the day together. It takes place the day before Mother's Day, so if you have a mom to celebrate, it won't interfere. At the brunch, attendees can enjoy a beautiful catered gourmet menu, swag bags filled with items from businesses that support the mission, and curated connection activities so women leave with new friends or an afternoon full of engaging conversation.

Since its inception in 2022, The Other's Day Brunch has grown. I've been invited to speak to news outlets and talk shows to spread the word. If you're reading this and thinking, *Wow! I want to be part of this*, join me! Women fly into Chicago from all over the world to be part of the connection that is created at this wonderful celebration. You can learn more about The Other's Day Brunch, reserve your spot for the upcoming celebration, or just reach out for more information by visiting lanamanikowski.com/othersday.

For your paper thinking today, I'd like you to take the opportunity to write an Other's Day card to yourself. What will it say about the awesome woman you are? What will it say about the loving person you are, who brings beauty and joy into the lives of others despite not being a mom?

25

Father's Day

As women without children, our lives can be filled with a lot of emotion. Sometimes, we get so lost in our own thoughts and feelings we may neglect to consider how our childlessness may be impacting the most important person in our lives—our partners. Mother's Day can feel like a black hole on the calendar, waiting for us to fall into it once a year. But what about Father's Day and how it impacts the men in our lives?

In years past, as Father's Day approached, I never really stopped to consider how Jack might be feeling. Both of us still have our fathers, and we're lucky enough that they are nearby and actively engaged in our lives. I've always associated Father's Day with my father and father-in-law and considered it a celebratory day because it simply doesn't impact me in the same way Mother's Day does. There are ways to offer support to the men in our lives, and I'd like to take this chapter to share some ideas that I've found helpful in my own marriage.

In many cultures and societies, men are often socialized to not speak of their emotions. In fact, observational research has shown that parents use more emotion-based language when speaking with their daughters than their sons, which leads to an increase in girls' expression of emotion and a decrease for boys. Jack does not talk much about how he feels about not being a dad. There have been a few instances when he has opened up and shared emotion or sadness around our situation, but it isn't often, and it certainly isn't at the rate I do! You may have a different dynamic with your partner, or the man in your life might be more open to speaking about his feelings. However, there are still plenty of things you can do to offer support to this person you hold so dear when Father's Day is looming on the calendar.

During our fertility treatments, it was rare for my husband to share feelings of sadness. He was aware of how much I was struggling through our fertility journey, and he wanted to be my rock and stay strong for me. In retrospect, I didn't recognize the sadness he may have been feeling. Maybe it's because I was the one with the infertility diagnosis, and I felt like it was all my fault and that my grief was more profound than his. I sometimes feel selfish for taking so long to recognize this but now that I have, Father's Day has taken on a new focus for us.

When Father's Day is coming up, I ask how he is feeling going into the weekend and inquire if there is anything special he may want to do—either together or by himself. I open the conversation to whatever he feels like doing, and then I agree to it. It's compassionate to bring up the topic and let our partners know we're supporting them too. If they're not into sharing much, that should be respected as well.

If your spouse isn't one to share, remind them that you love them and that you are here for them. The two phrases, "I love you" and "I'm glad we have each other," are so powerful. They really allow us to support people in whatever way they are looking to be supported. They are also useful phrases if your spouse doesn't want or need special treatment around Father's Day. Recognition for them might look like a peaceful, quiet afternoon at home rather than an event or outing of some sort. Letting them know that you love them and are here for them with open, acknowledging phrases gives them the space they deserve.

One thing I've started doing for Jack is getting him a Father's Day card from Coco, our dog. In the past, I've also gotten him a Father's Day card just telling him that I love him and reminding him of all the qualities about him that I admire as his wife. Last year we had a great breakfast and then went for a walk and got some exercise together on Father's Day morning. Because we both have our dads and I have a brother-in-law (the father of my niece and nephew), we'll sometimes plan a gathering of some sort, usually a brunch that we prepare at our place.

When I think about Mother's Day and everything we talked about that comes along with that—banners and specials and advertising—I have to consider that maybe Jack sees those same things around Father's Day but doesn't feel validated to talk about it. Being supportive and letting your partner know that you're thinking about them is a great way to allow them to communicate, if they feel like sharing.

So, when Father's Day comes around again, it can be a perfect time to be supportive to our partners. Let's ask them what they need and let them know that they are special and meaningful in our lives. Share with them the qualities you love about them, and although they don't have a child to share their talents and meaningful attributes with, they bring so much into the world just by showing up every day. Let them know they are celebrated and supported in whatever way they are willing to receive it.

For your paper thinking, take a moment to sit down and think about ways you can approach the topic of Father's Day with your partner. You know your man best! Is he someone who would open up and talk about his feelings, given the opportunity? Or would he react better if you showed him your love and support through nonverbal ways, like making his favorite meal or getting him a card and leaving it somewhere he can read it in private?

Remember to keep your partner and his needs in mind as this important date approaches on the calendar. Just as it is never too late for you to discover your meaning as an individual, strong, powerful woman, it's never too late to let him know he has the same opportunities as well—and you have an amazing chance to move forward in life together as a healthy, functioning couple who cares for and supports one another.

26

Birthdays and New Year's

There are a couple of dates on the calendar when it seems we are called upon to take stock of our lives—where you've been, what you've accomplished, what you desire, and what you're aspiring to achieve in the coming year. When you are childless after infertility it can feel suffocating to take an inventory like this. When life turns out so differently from what you expected, knowing what's next and where you want to go can feel challenging. It seems like nothing can compare to the life you dreamed of. Many of my clients struggle with moments of self-reflection at two particular times on the calendar—birthdays and around the close of a calendar year and the start of a new one.

Celebrating your birthday can come with different connotations as you age, particularly when you are a woman navigating IVF or have come to the realization that you won't have a biological child. So many women carry the hope that they'll be one of the miracle stories of a woman who went through years of treatment, only to conceive naturally after they "stopped trying." But our birthdays remind us of the ticking of the biological clock and all the pressures that come with it. Common things that come up for my clients around their birthdays are feelings of defeat, panic, disappointment, and confusion about what's next.

We know that birthdays are going to happen every year, yet there's a lot of anxiety about them. This doesn't have to be the case! Instead, let's focus on the freedom you can create in your life. You *can* be more connected to who you are and how you want to feel when that date on the calendar comes knocking each year. You may think your future as a woman without children will be a constant struggle, one where you are only making the best of it. But I've come to learn that there are tools to help me fall back in love with my life so that I can feel connected to it both now and in the future.

I have come to a point in my journey where I'm capable of deciding whether the thoughts and feelings that come up surrounding my birthday are the ones I want to surround myself with and whether they are going to help propel me into the future I am looking to create. There is such a sense of liberty I've come to feel about my birthday—even though it falls so close to Mother's Day. I've learned to utilize tools through life coaching that have allowed me to no longer dread getting older. Now I know that I can create a life for myself that I feel connected to, even though it turned out so differently than I thought it would.

New Year's is similar to birthdays in that we often think about things we would like to achieve or goals that perhaps didn't come to fruition over the last year. A lot of it has to do with goals you have for yourself versus expectations about what you think you should be doing. When you have goals, you give yourself the ability to dream about what you want and then create a plan or a roadmap to help you achieve it. Many women are conditioned to view certain expectations, like having children, as part of their identity simply because of their gender. This can shift the idea of having children from being a personal goal—one you feel a true connection with—to an assumed expectation. When the line between personal goals and societal expectations is blurred, it can create a sense of pressure and confusion around what you should be reaching for in your life.

Expectations are problematic because they're not always something you are choosing for yourself; they are commonly things society, family, or religion expect you to do to fulfill your role as a female. Expectations can generate frustration when you feel you aren't performing up to the demands of others. When we have that frustration, it interferes with the optimal results we want to achieve and can become part of a downward cycle of self-judgment that impacts how we show up in our lives, as well as the thoughts and feelings we carry.

One of the biggest mistakes I see childless women make is when they become set on a goal and put blinders on until they achieve it. It's what you think you're supposed to do—stop at nothing to achieve your goals—which may work until circumstances happen in your life that are out of your control. As hard as you've tried and as diligent as you have been about "doing what's right" or following your protocols, being a biological mother may not be part of your life journey. Learning to provide yourself the liberty of modifying your goals based on new realizations may allow you to reset what you want to be in life and, therefore, your goals as well. Thinking about your goal of motherhood in that way may open you to making modifications based on where you are now. Goals are *wants* not *needs*.

Navigating the new year can be particularly overwhelming for women who are childless after infertility. Throughout the year, there's often a reflection on how time has passed without the fulfillment of their desired parenthood journey. This reflection can lead to a sense of being stuck in a holding pattern, waiting for a clear direction or an aha moment to start shaping a new path forward in their childless life. However, without a definitive sign or direction, yet another year passes where you feel idle and uncertain about what comes next.

As the calendar turns to a new year, there's a societal pressure to set ambitious goals and resolutions. For childless women, there's a conflict between feeling compelled to declare these goals and not having the necessary support or plan to achieve them. This can lead to setting unrealistic expectations and ultimately feeling forced into the process, which only leads you to feeling disconnected from these goals. The lack of tools and support tailored to your journey as a woman who is childless after infertility can contribute to this sense of disconnect and difficulty.

I teach my clients how to feel more connected to the goals they choose—goals that are intentionally selected by you, for you, and based on your current understanding of what's available to you. This shift means no longer chasing what you think others expect of you. Instead, as you gain clarity about what truly motivates your desires and dreams, you'll discover how to thrive and feel fulfilled, even without the children you once envisioned. There is such freedom when you learn how to stop judging yourself for what has not happened in your life. It is such a relief to stop comparing yourself to others and dropping the shame you might be carrying about what you've encountered in your past. Right now, you're probably wondering how you'll ever get back to that point in your life where you actually love who you are and love the life you're living.

Let's start with your paper thinking. Make a list of all the things you have done since your last birthday or since January 1. These don't have to be earth-shattering achievements. Maybe you started working out two days a week, food planning, listening to a podcast, or reading more. Maybe you tried new recipes or started connecting with more childless women in your area. We give so much away when it comes to recognizing ourselves and our achievements—especially on a birthday or at New Year's. Often, we let the feelings of disappointment of not having yet achieved a certain goal overshadow the things that we *have* accomplished. So take a moment to really see yourself and the commitments you have made, no matter how small.

Now, take a moment and list all the things you would like to do *less* of before your next birthday or in the new year. Maybe you want to do less scrolling on social media, cut back on alcohol intake, or spend less of your personal time doing work outside of the office. Then, consider some things you would like to do *more* of. Maybe you'd like to set an intention to spend a certain amount of time outside each week, read a certain number of books in the next year, or get more face time with the people you love or friends you've not seen enough of lately.

Once you have your list, you'll be able to really see what you are already doing that is worth celebrating and what you'd like to do more of to help create a future you feel connected to. When you take the time to recognize that you are already accomplishing so much, you will develop a sense of pride in yourself. If you are like me, you'll never be a biological mother. But making a list like this shows that it was not another year wasted, that the next 365 days don't have to be full of feelings of defeat. You are doing amazing things despite not being a mom!

When you identify what you want to do more or less of, you'll have discovered a foundation for setting goals that doesn't revolve around motherhood. It is well within your grasp to lead a life that is fulfilling, one that you're connected to. You can live a life of growth, one with results you desire when you set your sights on goals of your own choosing that will enable you to remain flexible and avoid expectations.

So let's decide now that, despite not becoming a mom, you are already adding so much value to the world. Being unable to achieve your goal of motherhood does not mean your life cannot be full of meaning, full of purpose, and full of joy. You are a strong, capable, valuable human being who continually makes significant impacts each day. No matter what the date on the calendar is, it's never too late to recognize your value!

27

Baby Shower Invites

Whether it's preparing yourself to face a grocery store filled with Mother's Day banners and displays or bracing for the inevitable icebreaker questions about your motherhood status at social gatherings, finding ways to stay emotionally grounded is key to navigating moments that feel especially triggering. But sometimes, out of the blue, we are confronted with situations we weren't expecting, and it feels like "when it rains, it pours."

You've been managing everything pretty well, feeling like you are making progress with this hopeful outlook on your future, finding points of connection to a life that is so different from the one you thought you would have, and learning how to move through your days without being overwhelmed around every corner. And then, suddenly there's an invitation to a baby shower in your mailbox, and you're taken off guard—even though it's been obvious for many months that people around you are expecting.

The invitation feels like a total slap in the face. You may feel violated for being put in this situation—maybe even misunderstood—and it's likely you won't want to attend a celebration that feels like a dagger aimed for your heart. I've been there, and I've judged myself for feeling all these things. You may think you're not a good friend or that other people are going to believe you are jealous if you don't attend. You're worried that you might appear weak or that others will think you are self-absorbed because you can't put your sadness aside for one afternoon to celebrate someone else. So let's just decide right now that whatever you're feeling, you're entitled to feel it. It can be hard to celebrate something you wanted so badly and never will have. It can be exhausting to show up somewhere as an actor, out of fear someone will judge you.

I'd like to share some strategies that have worked for me when navigating baby showers. Whether you decide to attend or not, I hope these ideas will be helpful to you. You might be somebody who will show up even if you don't want to, and if that's the case, let's talk about ways to prepare yourself, even if you're not feeling super festive about the event.

One of the greatest things you can do to support yourself at an event like this is to make a plan before you go. Think about the event from start to finish and then section it out in chunks of time. Start with the first chunk as simply going to the shower. You show up, and maybe you drop off your gift and say a quick hello. Check in with yourself. How do you feel? Is it too much for you? If so, give yourself permission to leave. But maybe once you're there, you find you've got a little more gas in your tank than you thought, so you can stay for appetizers or the social hour and then do a quick check-in with yourself. See how you feel after that. If you want to stick around, that's awesome! If you don't, you can decide ahead of time that when it gets to be too much, you'll make your exit if that's what you need. But maybe you've got the endurance to stay for presents, perhaps even the dessert, right up until the other guests are leaving.

The most important thing is to have a plan and decide when to check in with yourself throughout the event. By doing this, you've created a sense of safety for yourself. You've got your own back. You've already thought this through, and any number of women in the infertility community—myself included—are right there with you if you decide to get in your car and go home at any point.

But maybe you're just not there yet. Maybe you got that invite, and you've decided to sit this one out. Let's talk about how to tell someone that you can't attend—you can do it or you may ask someone close to you to deliver that news on your behalf. This is complex; some invitations may hit harder than others so only do what you can. However you want to deliver the message, remind yourself that it's not coming from a place of jealousy or ill will, but from a place of love and acknowledgment for what you need and what you are capable of handling at this time.

If you are the one who is going to pick up the phone and call the mom-to-be, think about how you want that conversation to go. Write it down. Practice the delivery a few times. Remind yourself that the person who invited you loves you. If you've shared with this person about your fertility struggles, they know your not being able to attend the shower has nothing to do with them. They know you are working through complex things and are trying to preserve yourself for what you can shoulder at this time—and maybe this shower isn't it.

It's always possible that your declining the invitation won't be understood as you intended. That's okay. They may not realize the roller coaster you've been on through infertility. They've never known what it's like to spend a lifetime thinking you would be a mom and not be able to. If that's the case, they may not fully resonate, but what's most important is that you don't turn your back on your needs. If someone doesn't understand your absence, try to practice love toward this person. Revisit chapter 16, about acknowledging change in ongoing relationships, to help you navigate this situation.

Remember, the most important element here is for you to

support your needs and create a plan ahead of time. Do it from a place of love for yourself and preservation for your energy and emotional well-being. That is what is paramount right now. You may judge yourself for potentially disappointing a friend or not showing up for them on a day that is special to them. But things like that happen when you're navigating this unexpected path, and that's okay.

Own the road, and if you feel like you could use some support thinking through this, consider reaching out to someone you're connected with who gets it. Maybe its someone on social media who is childless after infertility. Reach out to me—I'll always be happy to talk through these types of scenarios. I will be happy to remind you that you're understood, welcome, and loved. I love you so much! You're so amazing and brave. I know that you're out there doing the best you can, every day. I see my clients and women in the communities I lead doing it all the time. They've realized it's paramount to put their own needs ahead of anything else—you can do so too. I believe in you!

28

Locations Associated with High Emotion

Oh, the places you *used* to go!

Have you ever found yourself avoiding certain locations because you associate them with your infertility? I know people who drive the long way home to avoid passing their doctor's office or fertility clinic; seeing a building that once loomed so large in their life is very triggering. It's one more instance where the outside world—your daily environment—can bring up something you weren't expecting. Unlike dates on the calendar or a planned event, these are feelings and situations that can take you by surprise and derail your day if you don't have a plan for how you face them.

Sometimes the place—like the waiting room in your OB/GYN's office—is pretty self-explanatory, and you don't have to do a lot of work to figure out why it holds so much emotion for you. But others might not be so obvious. I've felt triggers in places that I never anticipated, like the uneasiness that crept into my thoughts when passing the public restroom I'd duck into to give myself a MENOPUR shot. Going to the opera reminded me of the time I was in the bathroom during intermission and discovered that my period had started and my transfer didn't take. Standing in line at the pharmacy reminds me of the countless cycles I was stressing about because I wasn't sure they'd have all my medications available for me to start my protocol the next day.

Many of my clients feel like something is wrong with them when a wave of anxiousness hits them out of nowhere. For example, an uptick in emotion as you pull into the parking lot of your doctor's office because it's the same one where you parked your car for monitoring appointments and blood work countless times. It's common to feel overwhelmed or distraught when certain locations or types of places bring back intense emotions. This reaction can make you feel like you're losing your sense of control, but it's actually your brain's way of trying to protect you. These feelings often stem from the deep emotional challenges and anxiety you experienced during fertility treatments, and your mind is working to shield you from that pain.

So many things are sparked inside of us when we return to locations that once held so much connection to our journey of motherhood. When you learn to normalize that this is just what happens sometimes, you'll realize that it actually makes sense to have a surge of emotion or anxiety in these places because you're reminded of the panic you felt during your fertility journey. This realization can keep you questioning yourself, thinking that something is wrong or that your reaction is an overreaction.

You might pass judgment on yourself in that moment, thinking, *What is wrong with me?* You might even feel like you've reverted backward and are never going to get over this disappointment, all because catching a glimpse of Wanda in an exam room brings you to tears. You might be thinking that this feeling of being stuck is a representation of how broken you are—and how broken you will remain—for the rest of your life.

Let's think about whether this is the most supportive way to treat yourself, and instead consider this as something that is part of your process. What if every time you walk into the pharmacy and you feel triggered, you also take the time to have compassion for where you were then and then recognize where you are now? If you can start to note what places tend to raise strong emotion in you, you might create a dialogue with yourself that is supportive and compassionate while acknowledging the road you've been on.

At one time, I felt so helpless being here, but I survived. I am no longer navigating fertility treatments where I had no control over the outcome. My life is changing. I am changing too.

It doesn't mean you aren't healed if you react to being in certain locations. You may believe that no longer feeling such anxiety means you've come out on the other side. But if you still experience triggers and emotions you classify as negative, it must mean you haven't made enough progress in your life, right? But what if you take a moment and allow these things to coexist? Remember the woman you were back then and all the effort you gave to hold it all together. You made it through the days you didn't think you could. You did all those things, and you're still here today.

My advanced coaching certification in grief and post-traumatic growth has taught me that we may not ever be healed from something so challenging. We can't expect ourselves to never feel an emotion again. What we can do is feel an emotion without judging ourselves for having it. We can have compassion for it while recognizing how we are navigating through all of it.

The parking lot of my doctor's office and that bathroom stall aren't the only places that carry heavy emotion for me. As recently as a few months ago, I revisited the place where I got the voicemail from my reproductive endocrinologist delivering the results from genetic testing of my final (and only) frozen embryo. On that call, he shared that the embryo had trisomy 16 and would never lead to a viable pregnancy. That day I told you about in chapter 1—when I was hundreds of miles away from home, at a work event where most people didn't even know I was navigating fertility treatments. And here I recently was, standing within the very walls where I got the worst news I could possibly imagine. I became emotional. It played so vividly through my mind, like it was yesterday. I felt as though I could recount every step I took through those hallways after listening to that voicemail. Instead of judging myself for not being over it by now, I took a moment to talk myself through it. Many of the things I said to myself at that time will be helpful to you when you find yourself in a similar situation.

I know you weren't expecting to feel this way today. I know this still feels raw after all these years—that makes a lot of sense. But look at the commitments you've made to yourself. Look at how you've changed and grown. You are doing your best to create a life you love even though it did not end up with the children you always dreamed of.

I can help you learn how to stop judging yourself for being human and feeling emotions. You can feel more control. You have the ability to believe differently. I know it because you picked up this book, read this far. Maybe you visited me on YouTube or Instagram or have tuned in to my podcast. You wouldn't have done any of these things if you weren't somebody who's investing in a future that feels so much better and lighter than it did all those days, months, or even years ago.

For your paper thinking, take some time to notice and list what places have carried high emotion for you. What comes up for you when you find this happening? After that, acknowledge who you were then and list how you have changed and how you can experience that place now, as a compassionate, powerful, vibrant woman who is writing a new chapter in her book of life!

29

Owning Your Time

When you are faced with the reality that you won't be a mom, it's overwhelming to figure out how you will fill your time in a way that seems as meaningful and purposeful as you thought motherhood would be. If you spent your life thinking you would become a mom, then you likely viewed your future with milestones that mirrored those of raising a child. Your life was planned around the expectations of motherhood—helping with homework, driving to soccer games, prom, college visits, weddings, and eventually, becoming a grandmother. Now, without those milestones, your future may feel overwhelming and empty, like a blank canvas you didn't anticipate needing to fill yourself. The concept of how to meaningfully fill your time is so profound, it's one of the pillars of my coaching program, Thrive After Infertility.

Some parents may tell you not having kids is a blessing. Perhaps people with kids tell you how lucky you are to be able to do whatever you want, when you want. A mom may tell you that they'd love to trade places with you. To them, being able to go to a Saturday morning yoga class or drink their morning coffee on the patio uninterrupted seems like a luxury you're not appreciating. But having all this time to fill on your own isn't a comfort. Instead, it feels like a burden. There is a suffocating feeling that comes with realizing there is no predefined path.

You're left wondering what you will do with the next forty to fifty years of your life. You're asking yourself what can offer you the same sense of purpose, fulfillment, and meaning you expected from motherhood. By focusing on owning your time, this pillar will guide you through the process of figuring out how to create new milestones and experiences that bring joy and significance, helping you redefine what a fulfilling life looks like without children.

The realization that you will be the one responsible for filling the rest of your days can be overwhelming, but when we focus on this pillar in the Thrive After Infertility mastermind, we get clear on how to determine whether the things you are currently doing truly make you feel fulfilled. I'll help you determine if they will be part of the path that helps you create a life that feels meaningful and purposeful without children.

Through the work we do in Thrive After Infertility, most of my clients stop comparing their lives to those with kids because they become so connected to and fulfilled by the life they are discovering for themselves. They have gotten to a place where they see that they can create the life of their dreams without the children they always thought they would have. They are no longer dreading their future and worrying about growing old alone. It's a beautiful place to be, but it takes a curious heart to get there.

What I didn't realize at first was that I was being given an opportunity to dream a new dream, a chance to plan for a future I hadn't imagined, but one that still could be vibrant, joyful, and deeply meaningful. At first, I focused on small steps to reimagine myself and my future. The idea of crafting an entirely new life plan felt overwhelming, so I started with curiosity. I asked myself: *What interests me? How do I want to spend my time?* To my surprise, moments of peace would arrive unexpectedly, and I chose to lean into those moments, allowing them to guide me forward. I would ask myself: *Where am I when I feel such ease with myself? What am I doing that suddenly gave me this positivity and sense of calm?*

I started to pay attention to small moments, like sitting on a patio chair and listening to the birds, when I began to feel a sense of freedom or just the tension and stress of my life easing up a bit. Then, larger things began to happen when I put myself back in these places or situations that seemed to resonate with me. I found myself being creative again, becoming reinvested in activities I used to love and interested in new ones—like the idea to start my podcast and organize The Other's Day Brunch!

Pay attention to these moments and start finding ways to fill your time doing things that give you joy and peace. Be open to small steps in the beginning and then begin thinking about goals—any kind of goal. It could be financial, career related, the beginning of a new education, a relationship goal, or even a weight goal. By working with me in the Thrive After Infertility mastermind, I can help you determine what those goals might be.

When I gained weight during my fertility treatments—and three years later was still carrying around an extra twenty-five pounds and blaming the fertility medication for it—at what point was I going to stop giving away my power to my past? When was I going to acknowledge that yes, past Lana lost a connection to herself and her body, but Lana now (and future Lana!) had the option of turning her life around? For me, my weight loss journey started with understanding the relationship I created with food to soothe my loneliness. It gave me the opportunity to see that I can determine who I want to become so I feel connected to the future I want to create. It was the first step toward realizing that I have a say in my future, and I no longer want to think of myself as weak or broken.

Because I ended up childless not by choice, I didn't know

that a fully joyful and meaningful life was still possible. Even though I'm married to a wonderful man, and we have a great family and wonderful friends, and we do lovely things together, it always felt something was missing. It was as if I could only reach 80 percent happiness—like that remaining 20 percent was reserved for the fulfillment I thought only children could bring.

Achieving fulfillment without children once felt impossible to me. I now realize how damaging and suffocating that mindset was. I barely recognized myself anymore. I longed to reconnect with the woman I was before infertility—a woman who thrived in her career, embraced exciting and risky opportunities, and approached life with curiosity, confidence, and joy. I was fearless, outgoing, and eager to take anything on.

But somewhere along the way, I felt like I had given all of that up, losing my zest for life simply because I couldn't become a mom. If you're feeling this way, too, know that this doesn't have to be your reality forever.

If you're ready to dream about your future again and take steps to create a life you love, I'm here to help you. I know it's possible because I've done it myself, and supporting others in finding this fulfillment is my greatest passion. Learning to create a life I love—even though it looks so different from what I imagined—feels like I've uncovered a life-changing secret, and I just want to share it with the whole world! If you feel like it's your moment to step into a new future—one that feels fulfilling and purposeful—I can help you. Your first step is to book a free Thrive Call with me so we can start exploring how to create a life overflowing with meaning and possibility. If you've been searching for someone who understands where you've been and can guide you to where you want to go, that's exactly what I do. I'm here for you and ready to explore all the options that lie ahead.

If you're anything like me, you've probably spent time wondering what your legacy will be if you're not a mom. It's not something often discussed openly, but if you're part of online childless communities, my programs, or my circle, you know that defining a legacy is a significant hurdle for many women who are childless not by choice.

Your mind might race with questions about what the future holds. *What am I leaving behind? What mark have I made with my life? How will I be remembered?* These thoughts can feel overwhelming, especially when society has conditioned us to believe that raising children is the primary way to leave a legacy.

But here's the truth: Your legacy can be so much more than that. The belief that raising a human to create your legacy is limiting, and I've come to discover that a legacy is much bigger than that. It can include things like accomplishments, traditions, concepts and values, and maybe family history or heirlooms that are passed on to other family members through the years. Maybe you will be remembered as influential for all the contributions and lasting impacts you have made in your community and the lives of the people around you. Simple, everyday moments of kindness where you say hello, ask someone how they are doing, or offer a listening ear impart your legacy to someone. We've all experienced the unexpected beauty and kindness of other humans in everyday life, and for someone else, that may have been you!

Part of my legacy began when I created *The "So Now What?" Podcast*. I gave birth to—and continue to nourish—this impactful free resource that offers acknowledgment, awareness, and growth for anyone who wants to tune in. Sharing how to thrive in a life after IVF failed is my passion, and it's fulfilled me in a way I never knew was possible. Becoming a certified life coach for women who are childless after infertility offers me the amazing opportunity to impact the lives of other women who have been through this same struggle. This is a big part of the legacy that I will leave behind. Creating The Other's Day Brunch and bringing together and celebrating women who seek connection around Mother's Day will likely be part of my legacy. The many ways in which I've contributed to my family and how I live my life are part of my legacy and add to the fabric of our family story.

Now that you know your legacy is up to you to create, what will yours be?

You can start by asking yourself what you want to be known for. Do you want to be remembered as someone who sheds kindness on others? If that's the case, start saying hello to one stranger a day. They may not have anyone in their lives who fulfills that role for them, and it could make a huge impact.

Or give back by actively deciding to align yourself with a philanthropic organization or some sort of community service. Generosity through financial giving is always appreciated, but there are some lovely ways that you can be involved more directly by helping others, volunteering, or just showing up at a nursing home and participating in their activity hour. You can guide people or create opportunities to bring joy to your community, like joining an after-school program, starting a youth coloring club, or inquiring at your local rec center about what volunteer opportunities they already have in place. I guarantee there is so much uniqueness to you that can touch so many others through your greatness and the path that you have lived.

Something else that is important is documenting your journey. Consider keeping a record of your experiences, lessons you've learned, and accomplishments. We all have a story, we all have a journey, and very often we cut ourselves short by not recognizing everything we have encountered and accomplished. Things that happen in one moment can be forgotten in the next, so it's important to keep track of your life and make a record of it.

Family and friends may be a major part of your life, even when you don't have children of your own. What ripples are you creating when you genuinely show up as yourself with family and friends? See how you impact them and how they affect your life as well. If you have a desire to welcome new people in to your life, join a meet-up group or a book club. There are literally billions of people in the world who are waiting to meet you!

Sustainability is also an important thing to consider when thinking about your legacy. Maybe you'd like to impact the planet by cutting down on your use of plastic, recycling, and being more aware of your carbon footprint and energy usage. Someone once had me on their podcast, and she introduced me as an infertility activist. I never thought of myself as an activist, and hearing someone describe me in that manner felt so empowering. Find a cause that matters to you, champion a social issue that you're passionate about, and look for a place to leave your mark.

Leading by example is a beautiful way to accomplish this. Maybe it's by being a role model in how you live your life and how you have emerged from your infertility journey as a whole, transformed woman. You can be a positive example for people who may find themselves in the same situation one day. It's something that is a big driver in my life, and now I can impart motivation to others who find themselves childless not by choice.

Start to plan how you want to leave your matters in order as you age. We will inevitably accumulate money as well as possessions. Have a plan about where you want to leave what you have earned, making sure that your assets are distributed in a way that reflects your values and wishes. We may not be leaving things behind for our children, but there is so much we can give to a larger community.

Finally, know that just because you don't have kids does not mean you don't have a legacy. You have an option every day, the minute you put your feet on the floor, to create a legacy just by being yourself. Your legacy matters and can be impactful in so many ways, because you are impacting so many people. Our legacy as childless women can be so far- and wide-reaching. Know that your legacy matters.

As we reach the closing paragraphs of this book, I want to pause and express my deepest gratitude to you. Thank you for allowing me to walk beside you on this journey. Sharing my story is one of the greatest honors of my life, and my hope is that these words have brought you comfort, clarity, and the reassurance that you are not alone.

The path you've traveled is unlike any other—marked by dreams deferred, plans rewritten, and moments of deep reflection. But through it all, you've shown incredible resilience, even if it didn't always feel that way. Your courage to confront the unexpected and keep moving forward is a testament to your strength, even on the days you doubted yourself.

Writing this book has been an act of love—a love for the

woman you are and the life you are capable of creating. It's a love rooted in the belief that, even without the children you dreamed of, your life can be filled with immense joy, deep meaning, and unshakable fulfillment. I've walked this path, and while it wasn't always easy, I can say with certainty that it is possible to find light again. And I believe, with all my heart, that you can too.

You have the power to create a future that feels authentic and true to who you are, even though it looks different from what you once imagined. You've already taken the first steps by seeking out new possibilities and by daring to dream again. There is so much waiting for you—a world of experiences, connections, and moments that will take your breath away. You have everything within you to craft a life that feels vibrant and meaningful, one that honors your journey while embracing the beauty of what's to come.

As you move forward, remember to give yourself grace. This process isn't about rushing to the finish line or finding all the answers at once. It's about being gentle with yourself as you discover what makes your heart feel alive. Celebrate the small wins, lean into the moments of peace, and trust that the woman you are becoming is extraordinary in every way.

So, here's to the next chapter of your life—a chapter filled with hope, love, and fulfillment. Here's to dreaming new dreams, finding purpose in unexpected places, and building a life you feel connected to. You are worthy of all the beauty this world has to offer, and you deserve to feel joy and contentment in ways you never imagined.

With all my heart, I believe in you. You are stronger, braver, and more capable than you know. And while the journey ahead may still hold challenges, it will also hold so much possibility.

SO NOW WHAT?

The best is yet to come, and this is your time to embrace it.

With love and unwavering belief in you,

Lana

Resources

You can find a variety of resources on my website that will help you further implement the knowledge you've gathered from this book.

First, check out "The Top 27 Things People Say When You Are Childless (And How to Respond)" at: lanamanikowski.com/thingspeoplesay.

This free resource helps you feel more supported as you stumble upon awkward and unexpected scenarios where people ask invasive questions like: How many kids do you have? Why don't you adopt? This resource gives you suggestions for how to respond to flippant questions and suggestions and helps you manage those cringey moments.

Also available to you on my site is the "Learn to Love Your Life After Failed IVF." Find it at: lanamanikowski.com/guide.

Wishing there was a way to love your life again even though your dreams of becoming a mom didn't happen? It's possible to love your life, even if you're not a mother! I can show you how. The "Learn to Love Your Life After Failed IVF" guide is a workbook that helps you rethink the way you feel about creating a future you actually love, even without children.

And don't miss "Learn to Create Meaningful Holidays Even Without Children." Download it from lanamanikowski.com/holiday so you can learn how to start cherishing the holiday season again. This guide will help you start to feel connected to the holidays and enjoy this special time of year. Feel in control and supported this holiday season.

Whether you'd like to schedule a free Thrive call with me, listen to the podcast, attend The Other's Day Brunch, or join the Childless and Childfree Meetup group, there are so many ways we can stay in touch and support each other!

Website: lanamanikowski.com

The Other's Day Brunch: lanamanikowski.com/othersday

The "So Now What?" Podcast: available on Apple Podcasts and Spotify

Book your free Thrive call: lanamanikowski.com/thrivecall

Childless and Childfree Meetup group: meetup.com/childless-or-childfree-women

YouTube: @lana.manikowski

Instagram: @lana.manikowski

TikTok: @lana.manikowski

About the Author

Lana Manikowski is a certified life coach and advocate for women navigating life after infertility. With an advanced certification in grief and post-traumatic growth, Lana combines her professional expertise with her personal journey to support women in rediscovering joy, meaning, and fulfillment, even when life unfolds differently than they had planned.

After a seven-year fertility journey that ended without a child—and realizing that donor egg and adoption weren't the right paths for her—Lana was struck by the lack of resources for women facing a childless future. Determined to create the support she wished she had, Lana launched *The "So Now What?" Podcast* and her signature event, The Other's Day Brunch, an annual celebration for women without children held the day before Mother's Day.

Through her coaching practice, Lana helps women reconnect with themselves, build meaningful relationships, and create new milestones and experiences to fill the next chapters of their lives with purpose and joy. Her signature coaching program, Thrive After Infertility, guides women toward redefining what it means to thrive without the traditional milestones of motherhood, offering a path to a fulfilling, purposeful life.

Lana's insights have been featured in national media outlets, where she speaks openly about the unique grief of leaving fertility treatments without a child and the possibility of building a vibrant future. She serves as a living example that life after infertility can be both meaningful and deeply rewarding.

Lana lives in downtown Chicago with her husband and their beloved dog, Coco.

www.ingramcontent.com/pod-product-compliance
Ingram Content Group UK Ltd.
Pitfield, Milton Keynes, MK11 3LW, UK
UKHW030930230425
5581UKWH00021B/173